AWAKEN THE ABS WITHIN

7 Secrets To Lose Belly Fat

BRAD GOUTHRO, CPT & NWS

DEDICATION

Dedicated to my beautiful wife Kathy. I have a hard time expressing with words what your support, inspiration, and companionship throughout this journey means to me. You are my everything.

CONTENTS

ACKNOWLEDGMENTS

Thank you to my parents for raising me with a set of core values that has made me the man I am today. Your unconditional love means the world to me.

Thank you to Sherril Inglis Photography for providing the incredible cover photo.

GET YOUR FREE BONUSES NOW!

Get more **FREE BONUSES** such as:

"9 Steps to: Healthy Eating" &

"5 Abdominal Fat Burning Foods"

by visiting: **http://www.awakentheabswithin.com/free-stuff/**

FOR MORE RECIPES & WORKOUTS:

Join the Awaken The Abs Within Membership Site. Updated weekly with motivation and instruction videos, new healthy recipes, and workouts to get you ripped and lean.

http://www.awakentheabswithin.com/members

FOR MORE FITNESS & NUTRITION TIPS VISIT:

Blog: **http://www.awakentheabswithin.com**

Facebook: **http://www.facebook.com/bradgouthrofitness**

YouTube: **http://www.youtube.com/bradgouthrofitness**

Twitter: **http://www.twitter.com/bradgouthro**

MEDICAL DISCLAIMER

INTRODUCTION

Welcome to **Awaken the Abs Within**. My name is Brad Gouthro and I will be your coach, friend, and the positive/re-assuring voice in your head during this journey to a healthier, new you.

Before we get started, ask yourself these three questions:

- *Would you like to change the way you look and feel?*
- *Does all the conflicting information on fitness, nutrition, and health leave you so confused that you don't know where to start?*
- *Have you accepted your current health situation because it's the only way you know how to live?*

If you answered yes to one or all of these questions, this book was written for you.

It's time to put these negative thoughts and experiences in the past and realize you are not alone. Just look at these scary statistics:

o *Approximately 70% of Americans are considered overweight with 25% being visually and clinically obese. Every year the problem is getting worse.*

o *Based on the remaining 30% of the population that fall within the normal weight range, I'd take a guess that only 3-4% actually have VISIBLE abs.*

By purchasing and reading this book, you are demonstrating that you have the ability and motivation to be one of the 3-4% of the population with a flat stomach and sexy abs. So congratulations on taking the first step towards making a positive and healthy lifestyle change.

It's time to take ownership of your current health situation. Your lifestyle and dietary choices are far more important than the genes you were born with. Many scientists believe your lifestyle and the daily choices you make are responsible for 80% of your health status. This means your physical outcomes are mainly up to you. You can break the cycle and make positive changes if you choose. Remember, you and you alone, are solely in control of your health.

One of the main reasons people have so much trouble losing body fat is they do not specifically understand how they became fat in the first place. It is important to know how and why your body stores fat and how you can mobilize and use it as an energy source. With the wrong lifestyle, body fat constantly accumulates day-by-day and year-to-year. You don't go to sleep skinny and wake up the next morning fat. Fat piles on at a few ounces a month and eventually builds up and puts you on the trail to obesity.

If you are looking for effective and proven strategies to implement in your everyday lifestyle, than this is for you book. It will provide you with the necessary steps to burn unhealthy body fat and awaken the abs within.

I'd like to start this book off with one of my favorite quotes…

"Even the best workout program in the world can't correct stupid eating!"

As a certified fitness and nutrition professional, I've trained all kinds of different clients. Before I take on anyone new, I always mention this quote to make sure we are both clear on expectations. Some laugh, some frown, but most nod their head and agree. Awakening the abs within is 80% nutrition and 20% physical. Building six pack abs is more than just stressing the abdominal region with thousands of exercises. People need to clearly understand that *ABS ARE MADE IN THE KITCHEN, NOT IN THE GYM.*

If you only take away one thing from this book, I want it to be this…EAT WHOLE FOODS. If you never step foot in a gym or count a calorie, you will see noticeable changes to your belly fat by only consuming whole/real food. When I say whole foods, I'm referring to real food that has one ingredient. Examples are chicken, fish, turkey, veggies, fruit, and nuts. These are foods nature intended you to eat. More importantly, your body can properly digest and absorb the nutrients from these foods. THROW AWAY THE PACKAGED/REFINED JUNK! No more cookies, chips, crackers, ice cream, TV dinners, etc. A big part of this book is about understanding the affect certain foods have on your body's hormones. These hormones cause your body to BURN or STORE body fat. To control your hormones, it is as simple as eating the right types of foods, in the right quantities, at the right times. I've branded this as the TQT principle. We'll be discussing the TQT principle and hormones in more detail later.

Sexy abs are all about your lifestyle

The difference between this book and all the other ab books out there is this book focuses on the whys and hows of fat loss and conditioning. If you want to fix the problem (stored fat) you first need to understand how you got there. This book also discusses the necessary lifestyle changes that will cause you to drop the unnecessary body fat in an easy, simplistic, and understandable way. It's not just a short-term fix. This is a lifestyle change.

Most other books just give you an abs workout routine and a couple recipes. Not this book. This book is all about education and actionable steps. It's just like the Chinese proverb, *"Give a man a fish and he will eat for a day. Teach him how to fish and he will eat for a lifetime."* The Brad Gouthro proverb is, *"Give a person an abs routine and they will workout for a day. Teach them proper fitness and nutrition strategies and they will make health a lifestyle."* You need to understand how your body works in order to incorporate these 7 secrets into your daily lifestyle. This book will educate you with everything you need to know to awaken the abs within without being overly scientific or confusing. There are no gimmicks. You won't get six pack abs in five minutes. Once again, this is a lifestyle change. But I assure you, if you implement these 7 secrets into your daily lifestyle, you will see results.

I should mention up front…

Awaken the Abs Within IS NOT about:

- Providing you with a short-term 'fad diet' with outrageously restricted calorie counts that claims to make you lose 20 pounds in 1 week. Diets like this are not healthy and sustainable over the long-term.

- Eating the same boring, tasteless foods day after day.

- Telling you that you can never eat M&M's again.

- Instructing you to do 1,000 crunches every day.

- Giving you a generic abdominal routine and meal plan without any explanations.

Awaken the Abs Within <u>IS</u> about:

- Understanding that health, fitness, and nutrition is a lifestyle and not just something you pay attention to 6 weeks before your tropical vacation.

- Educating you on how to build a proper balanced nutrition plan that will fire up your metabolism, burn fat, and build lean muscle tissue.

- Understanding the macronutrients (protein, carbohydrates, fats) and their role in building muscle and burning fat (or adding fat).

- Understanding the important role your hormones play in establishing your body as either a fat-BURNING or fat-STORING machine.

- Providing you with a full body fat loss circuit and abdominal exercise plan that will condition, sculpt, and define the beach body everyone strives for.

Everyone has abs

It's true. You already have abs. I know it's hard to believe. So why can't you see them? Most people have a thick layer of body fat that hides the abdominal muscles. I can't stress this enough, you can do 10,000 crunches a day and still not see your abs if you continue to eat unhealthy food. As mentioned before, unveiling your abs is 80% related to diet and 20% related to the exercises in your workout routine.

A magical supplement pill cannot create six pack abs. The key to awakening the abs within is to reduce your belly fat levels and then strategically sculpt your abs with various exercises that target all areas of the abdominal region.

This book will uncover many ways to help reduce the stubborn stored fat by turning your body into a fat BURNING system rather than a fat STORING system. Not only will your confidence increase with your awakened abs, you'll also be creating a much healthier body. Abdominal fat is the most dangerous type of fat because of its close proximity to your body's vital organs. It can also create a lot of inflammation and destruction to the cells near by.

Before we go on, I need you to commit to changing your lifestyle for the better. It's not that hard. Just follow these secrets and you will see positive changes. Just think how much more confidence you'll have when you go to the beach. Think how much more energy you will have by losing the fat. You were born with two arms and two legs for a reason. You are supposed to use them to exercise! Exercise can literally be an addiction once you start seeing **results**. And that's what you're going to get by following this program.

I'll close this introduction with a quote from Albert Einstein:

> "Insanity is defined as doing the same thing over and over again and expecting different results."

Stop the insanity! Change your lifestyle. Change your habits. You know you need to make a change. You are responsible for your own health. Make the commitment. Don't accept anything less of yourself. You can do this.

One last thing. I want to ensure that you read this book from start to finish. DO NOT just skip the reading and go directly to the exercises. You need to understand how and why the body stores and burns fat. **Read first and then start the program.** Remember the Brad Gouthro proverb.

So what are we waiting for? I assume since you've read this far, you're ready to take the journey to awaken the abs within. Lets get started.

SECRET #1:

KNOW THY ENEMY (BODY FAT)

It's Time To Get Scared

Research shows it's more dangerous to be obese than to be a smoker. The health industry has come a long way in the battle to stop people from smoking cigarettes. In most public areas, you are not allowed to smoke indoors. They even designate certain areas outside where you're allowed to smoke. I personally love the new rules of making it an inconvenience for people to smoke. So what are we doing about obesity? How are we making it inconvenient for people to become obese? Most people would agree that we actually make it more convenient. Think fast food, instant microwavable meals, and vending machines in schools. These are all ways to instantly and conveniently become obese.

Here are a couple research findings on obesity that may surprise you:

- o Obese people have more chronic health problems than smokers.
- o In the US, there are more obese people than those who smoke, drink heavily, and live below the poverty line COMBINED!
- o Almost 300,000 North Americans die each year due to conditions attributed to obesity. That is approximately the entire population of Green Bay, Wisconsin.
- o In the US, 60% of people over 20 years old are carrying too much fat. Each year the problem gets worse.
- o Obesity costs US taxpayers approximately $100 billion a year.

Cardiovascular disease is the #1 killer in North America. Guess who is the prime target for this disease? That's right, the obese. Humans are becoming so fat that researchers are now saying obesity is outweighing the problem of starvation. What's even scarier is the youth of America are the first generation expected to have a shorter life span than their parents.

Death is the #2 fear that people have (behind public speaking). If we are so scared of death, why do we continually fuel our bodies with food that is making us obese? Next time you see a candy vending machine or fast food restaurant, become afraid.

Fat Fighting Misconceptions

Here are a few of the most common misconceptions (led by the diet industry and in some cases the government) to properly fight fat.

Misconception #1 – Focus on losing weight:

You will notice that I don't use the term 'weight-loss' throughout this book. Weight-loss is not a secret to awaken the abs within. Forget about using weight scales. It's all about body composition. Body weight is made up of many things, including muscle, fat, and stored water. Your goal to awaken the abs within should be about <u>FAT</u>-loss. You do not want to lose weight by losing muscle. As you will learn throughout this book, muscle is the metabolic driver that will keep the fat off. The rate of your metabolism is determined by the amount of lean muscle mass on your body. People that go on starvation diets may lose weight, but the real question is, where exactly is this weight-loss coming from? More than likely it's coming from lean muscle mass. When you lose lean muscle mass you're essentially becoming a smaller fat person. So from this point on, stop using the term <u>weight</u>-loss and start saying <u>fat</u>-loss.

Misconception #2 – Low fat foods will not produce body fat

Another common misconception is that the dietary fat in foods is the main contributor to excess body fat. Most dietary fat doesn't make you fat. Let me repeat. Most dietary fat doesn't make you fat. Don't be dietary fat phobic. In 1900, the average percent dietary fat consumption in the North American diet was close to 50%. Today it's about 32%. The American Heart Association actually calls a diet with 30% fat consumption a low fat diet. So why are we getting more obese every year when our dietary fat consumption is actually decreasing?

The truth is, you don't have to eat dietary fat to produce fat in the body. North Americans are now eating less fat than ever before, however the rate of obesity is still being doubled every 5 years. Did you ever notice that it's now hard to find full fat foods? Thirty years ago, food manufacturers started re-formulating food to create 'low fat' and 'no fat' food. It's interesting to note that after this happened, obesity rates skyrocketed by 50-60%. Re-formulated, low fat food is not the way nature built anything. Over consumption of sugar tends to be the main cause of obesity not dietary fat. Most of my clients have dropped the most amounts of excess body fat by eliminating refined sugar and reducing the consumption of grains from their diet. They focused on consuming carbs from fruits and veggies.

Just because you buy low fat food does not mean you will not produce excess body fat. Fighting fat is all about balancing your body's hormones. This is why one of the secrets to awaken the abs within is completely devoted to balancing your body's hormones. The human body has an amazing combination of hormones. These hormones are directly controlled by the nutrients you eat, the quality of exercise you participate in, and your lifestyle/environment. If your hormones are out of balance, your body has the ability to turn excess hormones, such as insulin, into excess body fat. More on hormones later. Don't fall into the 'Low Fat' label trap. If the label says it contains zero or small amounts of fat, it doesn't mean you can consume as much as you want and never gain body fat.

Misconception #3 – Combine a low calorie diet with excessive cardio to burn fat

To fight fat you must maintain muscle at all costs. Excessive cardio can actually inhibit fat loss because it can catabolize muscle tissue (note I said "excessive"). Muscle tissue is the key metabolic driver of the body. It can rev up thermogenesis, which incinerates calories to produce body heat. Fat is also shuttled into the engines of muscle tissue and burned for energy. The other great thing about lean muscle tissue is that muscles continue to burn fat even while resting. There are 3,500 calories in 1 pound of fat. When you add 1 pound of muscle, your body has the potential to burn 5 extra pounds of stored body fat per year. When you lose muscle, you lose this ability. It also takes more calories to move muscle than to move stored fat. For example, which person do you think would burn more calories by walking 5 miles at the same speed: a person with 40% stored body fat or a person with 8% stored body fat. The answer may surprise you. The person with more lean muscle mass would burn more calories than the "over fat" person. A proper BALANCE of cardio and resistance training is necessary for optimal fat loss.

Excessively low calorie diets are also the enemy of muscle. When you starve your body of calories and nutrients, a stress hormone is released to attack the muscle tissue to get energy. You need to feed your body a balance of good carbs (fiber), lean protein, and healthy fat to keep your body's hormones in balance, thus creating a fat BURNING system.

Your Body's Fat Cells

Your body has 100 trillion (yes trillion) cells. Approximately 30 billion of those cells store fat. 30 billion fat cells may seem like a lot but it only equals 0.03% of your overall cells. The tricky thing about your fat cells is they can expand 1,000 times their natural size and divide into more fat cells if you're not careful. On the flip side, if you make the necessary changes in your life, you can actually shrink your fat cells.

Did you know that some fat cells actually help burn stored body fat?

When most people hear the word fat, they usually think bad things. You need to realize that all fat isn't bad. Some fat actually plays a key role in your health and, interestingly enough, helps you burn fat.

Your body has two different kinds of fat cells. White andipose tissue (WAT) fat cells and Brown andipose tissue (BAT) fat cells. WAT fat cells create the unwanted excess body fat you love to hate. Your BAT fat cells do the opposite. Their function is to provide extra heat by burning body fat and creating thermogenesis. BAT fat cells are loaded with mitochondria (which are like motors) while WAT fat cells contain very little.

To simplify:

WAT Fat Cells = Hate

BAT Fat Cells = Love

Excess body fat can occur when your body has low levels of BAT fat cells or when these fat cells don't operate properly. Most people tend to have low levels of BAT fat cells, however some people are blessed with more active versions or just possess higher levels of these lovely cells. These tend to be the people who can eat anything they want and never gain body fat.

How do I create more BAT fat cells in my body?

The formula is simple. Exercise more and eat healthier. Doesn't everything health related always come back to that? By exercising and eating a healthy diet, your body mobilizes stored body fat and moves it to the BAT fat cells to be burned. Regular exercise and healthy eating also generates a more active thermogenic system in your body, which in turn can help generate more BAT fat cells.

The next time you complain about your body fat, make sure you direct your hate to Mr. WAT and share some love with Mr. BAT.

Comparing Fat Cells: Male vs. Female

If you're a female, you may be interested to know how your body's fat cells compare to your male counterparts. Before I go on, please remember the following is not to be used as excuses for why you may be over fat. Take the following as a challenge. Despite what you're about to read, I'm challenging you to set goals, overcome these hurdles, and experience the healthy body you were intended to have. To the guys, after reading this you will see how easy you have it compared to females. You have no excuses to be over fat.

Female fat cells:

- are 5 times larger than male fat cells.
- can contain up to twice the fat-STORING enzymes as male fat cells.
- can contain only half the fat-BURNING enzymes as male fat cells.

On top of all of this men:

- on average, carry 40 pounds more muscle (muscle helps burn fat) than women.
- produce 10 times more testosterone (helps burn fat) than women.
- can burn 30% more calories during exercise & at rest than women.

How fair does that sound? Because of this, it can be much easier for women to gain fat and much harder to burn fat than men.

Studies show women need at least 16% body fat to allow for proper hormone (childbearing needs) production. Healthy body fat % for women is 16-24%. Healthy body fat % for men is 6-17%.

Did you know: 99% of your genetic structure was formed more than 40,000 years ago?

40,000 years ago it was a feast or famine environment. Food wasn't always plentiful so our ancestors would eat as much food as possible when available and then store the extra calories as body fat. This stored body fat was their only way to survive during times of famine. Because of this, eventually our bodies became very good at converting most things into body fat. Even though most of us do not live in a feast or famine world anymore, our bodies still employ this fat hoarding tactic.

99% of your genetic structure was formed more than 40,000 years ago. Think about that for a second. Now think about the different foods people eat today compared to what your ancestors ate 40,000 years ago. Your genes control every function in your body. Therefore it's important to consume foods that are compatible with your genes. Look at it this way, we still have a Fred Flintstone body but are feeding it food from the George Jetson era. If you want to live a life free of excess stored body fat, start by focusing on the type of foods you're consuming. The majority of your food should come from whole, natural food that is free of manufactured additives, chemicals, and pesticides. These are the foods that are compatible with your genes.

If you look in the grocery cart of most people today you'll see a cart filled with refined/processed food. There is nothing natural about these refined foods. They are stripped of their nutrients and injected with preservatives and chemicals to increase shelf life.

Here's an easy tip while at the grocery store. Shop on the outer edges of the store. All the junk is found in the middle aisles. Also start paying attention to the ingredients label and stay away from any products that contain words that you cannot pronounce! These foods will be very unfamiliar to your body. Do you think your ancestors of 40,000 years ago ate Oreo cookies? These refined foods are foreign to your genes and your body does not know what to do with them when they are consumed.

Research shows our ancestors took in 500% more vitamins and minerals and 300% more fiber than today's diet. Genetically, your body was made for a diet consisting of lots of vegetables, a limited amount of fruit, lean meat and fish, nuts, legumes and seeds. Once again, refined carbohydrates and over processed fats are foreign to your genes.

Unfortunately, today's unhealthy diet focuses on carbohydrates as the meal's main food source rather than protein. Your ancestor's diets consisted of at least 30% from protein sources. An old study in the US reports that the average US diet consists of 46% carbohydrates, 43% fats (not the healthy ones), and only 11% protein. Today's diet ratios are probably worse. The body wasn't designed to use an incredible amount of carbohydrates for energy. The over consumption of carbohydrates in my opinion, is the leading cause of increasing obesity rates in North America.

The next time you are chowing down on a chocolate chip cookie, ask yourself if your ancestors were eating the same thing 40,000 years ago.

What's Your Current Body Fat %?

To get to where you want to be, you need to know where you currently are. As mentioned earlier, we do not want to measure body weight as our target for fat loss. Body composition, the percentage of weight coming from lean muscle tissue vs. body fat, is the method we want to focus on.

Body fat % is calculated as follows:

- Total body fat weight divided by total body weight

Your total fat calculation consists of your body's essential fat (the fat necessary to maintain life) and stored body fat. Some body fat is required for life. Here's an example of how to calculate the body fat % of a 172-pound person. If the 172-pound person carries 13.4 pounds of body fat, their body fat % would be calculated as follows:

- 13.4 pounds of body fat / 172 pounds total body weight = 7.8% body fat

A healthy man's body fat % should not exceed 17%. A healthy women's body fat % should be between 16-24%.

General Body Fat % Categories

Classification	Women (% fat)	Men (% fat)
Essential Fat	10-12 %	2-4%
Athletes	14-20%	6-13%
Healthy	21-24%	14-17%
Over-Fat	25-31%	18-25%
Obese	32%+	25%+

There are several ways to measure your body fat %, however the most reliable and cost effective measurement is with a bioelectrical impedance analysis (BIA) machine or measuring skin folds with a set of skin fold calipers by a trained individual.

Your fitness center should be able to provide you with this service for a fee.

Let's move on to learn more about one of the most important secrets. Your hormones.

SECRET #2:

CONTROL YOUR BODY'S HORMONES

What are Hormones?

Hormones are the tiny chemical messengers that control the overall communication within your body. Achieving hormonal harmony is such an important key to fat loss. Achieving hormonal harmony is the difference between living with a body that is a fat BURNING machine rather than a fat STORING machine. Which body would you prefer?

When most people talk about adding muscle or losing body fat, they investigate new muscle building programs and how to incorporate "low fat" foods into their diet. This is fine, but if you really want to turn your body into a fat burning and muscle-building machine, you must learn about your body's hormonal system! Having hormonal imbalances can also cause 'false fat' which can be an extra 10-15 pounds of <u>water weight</u> that is trapped in the tissues. This contributes to abdominal bloating, cellulite, and face and eye

25

puffiness. This is not true fat; it's just excess water. This hormonal imbalance is caused by your body producing too much of certain hormones based on the foods you are eating. Many of these foods may have been injected with fattening hormones. To get the six pack/flat stomach look, you need to ensure your hormones are balanced so you're not holding onto unnecessary water weight that is trapped between the muscles and the skin. This will put a halt on all progress towards looking ripped.

Your Phenotype

Your genotype (genes) is fixed. As mentioned earlier, you have 99% of the same genes as your ancestors from 40,000 years ago. The part you can control is your phenotype. Your phenotype is the expression of your genes and is directly influenced by the foods you eat, your environment, and your lifestyle. This means your phenotype is controlled by YOUR actions. The food you consume, the exercise you do, and the amounts of rest you get, all stimulate your hormonal system to send fat BURNING or fat STORING messages to your body. No matter how much you exercise, if your body's hormones are out of sorts, your body will turn itself into a fat storing machine. It's absolutely amazing how much responsibility your hormones have on your body cells.

Your body has nearly 30 hormones at work. Only a few of these are involved in the fat gain or fat loss process.

Within this section the following main hormones will be profiled:

- Insulin
- Glucagon
- Human Growth Hormone (HGH) & Albumin

- Testosterone
- Cortisol

Before we profile each hormone, lets do a little comparison to show you how different foods impact your body's hormones.

Today's typical meal vs. a meal you were actually intended to eat

Unfortunately in today's society it has become 'normal' to have bad nutrition habits. The odd balls have become the people who consume 5-6 macronutrient balanced (protein, carbs, fats) meals per day, are in control of their sugar cravings, and are oddly enough, healthy.

Below is a step-by-step comparison of how the body and its hormones react based on today's typical meal vs. a meal you were actually intended to eat.

Today's Typical Meal

Here's what happens in your body when you consume today's typical refined carbohydrate meal (lets say a bowl of sugary cereal):

1. Once the cereal makes contact with the tongue, the tongue senses the sugar and initiates the release of endorphins causing a short-term sense of satisfaction, calmness, and euphoria. **The sugar enters the bloodstream very quickly.**

2. Since your blood can only handle a minimal amount of sugar in the blood, the pancreas releases a **large amount** of a hormone called insulin to help deal with the excess sugar (more on insulin later).

3. Insulin removes the excess sugar from the bloodstream and stores a limited amount as short-term energy in the form of glycogen in the

muscles and liver cells.

4.   In the meantime, a FAT STORING enzyme called LPL is stimulated by the release of insulin. The LPL enzyme converts the excess sugar that has not been used for immediate energy or stored as glycogen into **STORED BODY FAT** (at least 40%)!

5.   Since the sugar has been quickly removed from the bloodstream, your blood-sugar levels become very low which causes irritable and depressed feelings as well as sluggishness.

6.   To bring back the short-term sense of satisfaction, your body craves more sugar to raise blood sugar levels back up. Then the whole scenario repeats itself. Ever noticed you can't just eat one chip? This is why.

A Properly Balanced Meal

Now here's what happens in your body when you consume a properly balanced meal including high quality proteins, low glycemic carbs, and healthy fats:

1.   Once the sugar makes contact with the tongue, the tongue senses the sugar and releases endorphins making you feel good, calm and satisfied. The sugar and amino acids (from the protein) **slowly enter the bloodstream** including tryptophan (an initiator of the appetite control brain chemical serotonin).

2.   The pancreas releases a hormone called glucagon.

3.   A FAT BURNING enzyme called HSL is stimulated by the release of glucagon. HSL initiates the release of **FAT TO BE BURNED** as

a primary source of fuel (rather than being stored as body fat).

4.   Blood-sugar levels are now stabilized and **you're burning fat as a primary fuel source**. You also begin to feel energetic with a sense of well-being.

5.   Your hormones are properly balanced, you continue to burn fat for energy, and you feel full and satisfied for three to four hours.

This example is to show how nutrition affects your body's hormones. Lets look at each hormone in more detail.

INSULIN HORMONE: Controlling Your Insulin Levels By Kicking Sugar Out Of Your Life

What is Insulin?

Insulin is a hormone secreted immediately from your pancreas following consumption of a carbohydrate rich food. Insulin plays a key role in controlling the amount of sugar in the blood after you eat carbohydrates. It helps remove sugar from the blood stream and places a limited amount into the muscle and liver tissues in the form of glycogen. **Your glycogen storage levels are limited**. So when the muscle and liver glycogen storage levels are full, the excess sugar is converted to body fat with the assistance of insulin (i.e. the spillover effect – more on this later).

3 important things to remember about insulin:

1.   It stores fat

2.   It lowers blood sugar levels

3. It's triggered by carbohydrates

As you will learn, insulin can have positive and negative effects on the body. Without insulin you will die. However with excessive quantities of insulin, you will become obese. It all goes back to balance.

How Do I Balance Insulin?

To counteract the negative effects of insulin, it needs to be paired with the opposing hormone glucagon. Glucagon is released by the consumption of protein. We'll discuss glucagon in more detail in the next section. The glucagon hormone has the opposite effect of insulin on our bodies. It raises blood sugar levels and mobilizes fat from storage. This is why the combination of protein with carbohydrates is so important. It's also important to eat mainly unrefined carbohydrates and reduce the amount of refined/processed carbohydrates from your diet.

The Positive Side of Insulin

Insulin plays a major role in building muscle after a workout. After an intense workout, your muscles are broken down and your body is depleted of muscle glycogen (which puts your body in a catabolic state). By consuming a high glycemic carbohydrate after your workout, it creates an insulin spike. This insulin spike provides an excellent delivery system for the muscle glycogen and amino acids (protein) to reach the muscle cells. This helps re-build stronger and bigger muscles and replenishes your previously depleted muscle glycogen levels (bringing your body back into an anabolic state).

The Negative Side of Insulin

Insulin plays a negative role when produced in excess. It is a primary fat storage hormone. As mentioned earlier, when refined carbohydrates are consumed, they break down into sugar and quickly enter the bloodstream. A large amount of insulin is required to clear the sugar from the blood. At anytime, your entire bloodstream can only contain approximately 5g (a teaspoon) of blood sugar.

Now think about how a cinnamon roll, containing 60g of sugar, will affect your body's hormonal balance. Lets break this down.

60g of sugar quickly enters the bloodstream, thus a massive amount of insulin is required to remove the excess from the bloodstream. When you consume refined carbohydrates, 30% is burned as immediate energy, another 30% is stored as glycogen in your liver and muscle cells as short-term energy, and the remaining 40% is stored as long-term energy (body fat). As discussed earlier, insulin also releases the fat storing LPL enzyme. When this LPL is released, it has a mission to store everything as fat. Insulin causes most of the fat to be stored in the abdominal region (belly fat).

The Spillover Effect Example

Lets take another look at how a "low fat" cinnamon roll can really be a fat filled mess.

A cinnamon roll containing 60 grams of sugar will be broken down as follows:

1. 30% is burned as immediate energy (18g of sugar)

2. 30% is stored as glycogen and burned as short-term energy (when required) (18g of sugar)

a. Note: When required! This means if you're not exercising enough and your muscle and liver glycogen levels are already at capacity, there will be no room to store any more sugar as glycogen in your muscle and liver cells. Therefore, this 18 grams of sugar gets sent to step 3...

3. 40% is STORED AS FAT! (24g of sugar)

Here's something even scarier. As mentioned in number 2, your glycogen tank has a limited capacity to store short-term energy. So if your glycogen tank is already full, the following happens:

- 30% is burned as immediate energy (18g of sugar)

- 0% is stored as glycogen since the tank is already full (0g of sugar)

- 70% is STORED AS FAT! (42g of sugar)

This is what happens to people that don't exercise and continuously over indulge on sugary foods.

So next time you read a label that says the cinnamon rolls are low fat...think again.

Other Negatives About Insulin

Your body is designed to burn fat for 70% of its energy requirements. When you have high insulin levels, your body burns glucose and amino acids for energy rather than burning fat. Another negative affect of insulin is how it reacts with other fat burning agents. Carnitine is a compound in the body that helps shuttle fatty acids into your cells mitochondria to be burned as fuel. When insulin is in excess, it lowers the level of carnitine in the body, thus halting fat burn. Constant high insulin levels (caused by continuously consuming sugary foods and not exercising) causes the body to store sugar as body fat. It can also inhibit the future breakdown of stored body fat as fuel.

So how do you avoid this and keep your insulin levels low?

The key to long-term fat loss is balancing your insulin levels by consuming the right types of carbohydrates (unrefined, natural), in limited quantities, at the right times. This will be discussed in more detail along with a full list of the right types of carbs to eat in Secret #4 on Meal Planning. It's also about always consuming a protein source with carbohydrates and ensuring you're getting enough exercise. The higher your sugar consumption, the higher your insulin levels will be.

GLUCAGON HORMONE

The positive and negative role of the insulin hormone was discussed above. To quickly recap, insulin plays a positive role in the body when it is properly regulated. It removes blood sugar from the bloodstream and delivers glucose and amino acids into the cells. When large amounts of high glycemic, refined carbohydrates are consumed, you quickly receive an insulin hormonal imbalance that releases a fat storing enzyme called LPL. This enzyme literally turns your body into a FAT STORING machine.

The antagonist hormone to insulin is called glucagon. The glucagon hormone helps prevent low blood sugar levels. Low blood sugar levels occur when people follow low calorie diets, over exercise, and skip meals. Glucagon is stimulated by the consumption of quality protein. When glucagon is released, it produces a fat burning enzyme called HSL. Differing from LPL, the HSL enzyme turns your body into a FAT BURNING machine.

By keeping both insulin and glucagon in balance, your fat cells will deflate and your body will maintain its role in burning fat for energy rather than storing it.

Insulin sets the stage for fat gain, while glucagon sets the stage for fat loss. This is just another reason to cut sugar consumption from your diet. Replace sugary foods with low glycemic carbohydrates and eat a high quality protein source with every meal such as lean meat, chicken, fish, whey protein powder, or eggs.

HUMAN GROWTH HORMONE (HGH)

Human Growth Hormone (HGH) has received a lot of negative press the last few years due to athletes supplementing with illegal, unnatural hormones. With this negative press, some people may be unaware that HGH is actually produced in the body naturally (via the pituitary gland) and is a very important hormone for building lean muscle tissue and burning excess fat.

HGH's mission is to activate the release of stored fat for energy and release insulin-like growth factors (IGF) that assist in the growth of muscles, cells, and bones. Up to 75% of HGH is produced during sleep as well as during intense resistance training. Therefore, to take advantage of this natural hormone, you need to ensure you get adequate amounts of sleep and incorporate resistance training into your day. By staying up late, you can actually cut into how much HGH will be produced by your body. According to the below HGH Secretion Patterns, you should be in a deep sleep by 11pm in order to produce optimal levels of HGH. Also as you can see in the patterns below, your body secretes a high level of HGH at 12pm. Therefore this is a great time to schedule your intense resistance training workouts.

24-Hour HGH Secretion Patterns

7am – low secretion

9am – medium secretion

11am – low secretion

12pm – HIGH secretion (optimal intense resistance training time)

2-5pm – low/medium secretion peaks

7pm – medium/high secretion

12am – VERY HIGH (should be in a deep sleep by 11pm)

3-6am – small peaks

The Negative Effect Insulin has on HGH Secretion

When you consistently have high levels of insulin (from consuming large amounts of high glycemic, refined carbs), it negatively affects your body's anabolic response by lowering HGH levels. To efficiently produce HGH for muscle tissue growth and fat burn, it is very important to keep your insulin levels in balance.

HGH Secretion Declines As You Age

After your 20's, HGH declines by 14% per decade. By the age of 60 your HGH production declines by 80%. IGF (growth helpers) also declines by 50% after the age of 40. These declines strip you of your metabolically active lean muscle mass. This is why it's so crucial for aging males and females to include resistance training in their everyday lifestyle. It will help maintain muscle mass and keep you younger in the process.

DO NOT purchase HGH products that actually contain HGH unless prescribed by your physician.

Albumin

Albumin is a transport protein in the body that plays a major role in keeping the fat off. It transports fatty acids, nutrients, and removes waste from the body. To be blunt, it's very hard to be fat with high levels of albumin. The more albumin produced in the body, the healthier you'll be. With high levels of albumin, the blood can easily transport fat (including cholesterol) to be burned off rather than being stored.

Albumin Levels

Depending on your level of health, here is the amount albumin that should be found in your body:

- Average Person: 40g of Albumin/litre of blood

- Healthy Person: 50g of Albumin/litre of blood

- Super Healthy Person: 55g of Albumin/litre of blood

If you're interested in finding out more about your albumin levels, ask your physician for an Albumin count test.

How Can You Ensure Your Body Produces Lots of Albumin?

The greater the stress on your immune system, the lower your levels of albumin will be. High protein diets, supplements, and IV injections won't directly raise counts. Proper hygiene is the only way to raise albumin production. When your body detects germs, the liver reduces albumin production. This causes less fat to be mobilized. When your body is clear of germs, the liver produces more albumin, thus mobilizing fat. Focus most of your hygiene efforts on keeping hands and finger nails clean and keeping your hands away from your nasal passages, eyes, and mouth.

Another way to ensure optimal production of albumin is to fast (no solid food) from the evening (after supper) to the next morning. It's also essential to get plenty of sleep. While fasting and sleeping, your body produces optimal levels of albumin and HGH. Your supper should be no later than 8pm. By getting proper sleep and keeping your insulin levels low, the body will switch to fat burning mode during this time frame. If you need to eat at night, drink a protein shake mixed in water (no carbs).

TESTOSTERONE & ESTROGEN HORMONE

Think testosterone is just a sex hormone? WRONG.

Why Your Body Loves Testosterone (both males and females):

- Increases energy and stamina

- Lowers stress (i.e. the stress hormone Cortisol)

  - Burns excess body fat

- Assists proteins in building lean muscle mass (which helps burn fat)

- Improves oxygen uptake (oxygen helps burn fat)

- Helps control blood sugar/insulin levels

- Builds strong bones

After the age of 35, testosterone levels tend to decline in males. This decline can weaken muscle strength, bone matter, and can lead to increased levels of excess body fat storage. A good percentage of people with low testosterone levels have a higher BMI (body mass index) and higher body fat percentage. Studies also show people with higher levels of testosterone have higher levels of HDL (good cholesterol) and lower levels of LDL (bad cholesterol) and triglycerides (fat). Belly fat can be a signal that men are losing their testosterone levels.

Free Testosterone

Not all testosterone in the body is active. Only free testosterone is active. It's the free testosterone that is very important. Unfortunately free testosterone levels decline with age caused by a sex hormone-binding globulin (SHBG). Once the SHBG is bound, your free testosterone can no longer enhance muscle or burn fat. If you're worried about low free testosterone, consult your physician for a check up.

Raise Testosterone Levels

When testosterone levels drop in aging men, estrogen levels usually increase. Retirement aged men can actually have higher estrogen levels than women of the same age. As men age, they tend to lose muscle and gain fat. The fatter they are the higher the conversion of testosterone to estrogen. To help prevent this conversion, you can raise testosterone levels by performing strength resistance exercises to build more lean muscle mass and burn fat. Regular sex can also helps raise testosterone levels. Regular sex means 2-3 times per week. Research shows that men that have sex 2-3 per week live longer. For women, during sex, the hormone oxytocin (the bonding hormone) is released which helps lower women's cortisol levels i.e. the stress hormone. Remember, excess stress can lead to fat storage. So not only does a healthy sex life help burn calories, it also can increase the release of hormones that help keep the fat off.

Hormone (Estrogen) Injected Meat – STAY AWAY!

Some farmers are putting estrogen (a fat storing hormone) in their livestock to produce fatter (more profitable) poultry and meat. When humans eat this meat, the estrogen also gets transferred into our systems. These unnatural hormones can lower testosterone (the fat burning hormone) and increase estrogen (the fat storing hormone) in your body. This is just another reason to try to eat organic (non-hormone injected) meat and poultry.

CORTISOL

Ways To Reduce Cortisol (Stress hormone)

Cortisol is a hormone that is produced by the body in times of stress. Stress not only strips your body of muscle (the metabolic engine) but can also cause your body to store fat and prematurely age your body. Here are a few tips to reduce the stress in your life (more on positive thinking later in the book).

1. Hang out with positive people.
    - A study using 30 test subjects found that cortisol production was reduced by 23% just by thinking more positively.
    - Stay away from people that are creating stress in your life

2. Incorporate more stress reducing activities in your day.
    - Yoga, Bike Rides, Surfing, and Meditation.

3. Focus on what you have control over.

   • Forget about what is out of your hands.

4. Live in the now.

   • Forget about what happened in the past.

5. Know when to say no.

   • You can't be everything to everyone. Don't be a people pleaser. If you don't first take care of yourself, you won't be able to take care of anyone else.

Isn't it amazing how powerful hormones are? What's even more amazing is we are in control of how these hormones react within our body. Your day-to-day nutrition has a big impact on these hormones. More on nutrition in Secret #3.

SECRET #3:

TQT PRINCIPLE TO MEAL PLAN DESIGN

Contrary to popular believe, portion sizes haven't actually grown as much as you may think. Although the supersized fast food meals are contributing to the obesity epidemic, excessive caloric intake is not the main reason for us becoming fat. As you know, in order to lose fat, you need to create a caloric deficit. Essentially burn more calories than you take in. That may sound simple. But not all calories are created equally. Do you think eating 100 calories of broccoli has the same affect on your body fat as 100 calories of ice cream? Think again. Since the 1970's, the calories we eat per meal has not changed that much. What has changed is the composition of the macronutrients in the meal (proteins vs. carbs vs. fats). The composition of the nutrients impacts how your body uses fat for energy. The type of food, and when you consume it, has a major impact whether your body STORES fat or BURNS fat for energy.

To properly burn body fat and build muscle, you need to feed your muscles the right **T**ypes of food, in the right **Q**uantity, at the right **T**imes. I've branded this the **TQT Principle**.

In this secret it's important to learn about the macronutrients that make up the calories you eat throughout the day and how to use them to create a balanced meal plan. The role of the micronutrients will also be discussed. **<u>All 7 secrets in this book are important, however this step is one of, if not, the most important to understand.</u>**

The 3 Macronutrients

When you hear the word macronutrient, don't be afraid. It's a long word that is used to explain a simple thing:

- o Macronutrients equal:
  - o Proteins
  - o Carbohydrates
  - o Fats
- o Micronutrients equal:
  - o Vitamins
  - o Minerals
  - o Water

All of these macro and micronutrients are essential to your health and building the body you've always wanted. However, consuming as many or as little of each nutrient as you want will not give you the results you're looking for.

To reach your goals you need a strategic plan that outlines:

- o **T** - The right **Types** of protein/carbs/fats to eat
- o **Q** – The right **Quantity** of protein/carbs/fats to eat
- o **T** – The right **Times** to eat the protein/carbs/fats

This is what the TQT Principle provides.

Lets start with the first T in TQT. Type.

Types of Food

There are good and bad sources of Protein, Carbohydrates, and Fat. In order to reach your goals, you need to focus on the right **TYPES**.

Protein

The word protein comes from the Greek word "proteis". It means 'of prime importance'. Makes sense doesn't it? Besides water, protein makes up the largest percentage of material in the human body (45%). This is why, starting today, protein is now the central theme of your meal plan. Always build **ALL** your meals/snacks around a protein source. When you're thinking of what to eat, you should immediately ask yourself what lean source of protein do I want to eat? It may not be the norm to you now, but it will soon become the norm when you start seeing the results. Start with protein and then add the other macronutrients to your meal.

As mentioned earlier, the term 'false fat' refers to excessive water that is retained in the body for no good reason. When the body is deficient in protein, stored water fluid can leak from the vascular spaces between the cells and can become trapped. This causes sagging and dragging of the tissues, called cellulite.

Protein can have a great impact on reducing the false fat by attracting the stored water molecules and shuttling them through the kidneys where it is removed. Protein is very water loving. By eating protein during every meal and snack you can help rid your body of the 'false fat'.

Protein is very thermogenically active, meaning your body burns a lot of calories during digestion of the protein source. It also increases production of good chemicals in the brain (dopamine and serotonin) and cuts down on your appetite as it makes you feel fuller.

There are 4 calories in 1 gram of protein.

Amino Acids – The Building Blocks of Protein:

Protein is comprised of amino acids. Amino acids are often referred to as the building blocks of protein. Visualize protein as a chain-link fence. Each link in the fence is considered an amino acid.

There are 21 different amino acids that make up protein. The human body is capable of producing 12 non-essential amino acids (this is why they're called non-essential). The remaining 9 are called essential amino acids because the body cannot produce them on it's own. You must get these amino acids from food sources.

It's important to focus on complete protein sources that contain all 9 essential amino acids in proper proportion. The nutritional label on a package may say the food contains protein but the food may not have all the essential amino acids (or the right amount) that will provide your body with the most important muscle building benefits. This is just another reason to learn and focus on eating the right TYPES of protein. A full list of excellent sources of protein will be listed shortly.

Although you don't need to know every amino acid, it still may help to have a list of the essential and non-essential kinds for reference.

9 Essential Amino Acids (must be obtained via food)		
Histidine	Isoleucine	Leucine
Lysine	Methionine	Phenylalanine
Threonine	Tryptophane	Valine

12 Non-Essential Amino Acids (produced by the body)		
Alanine	Arginine	Asparagine
Aspartic Acid	Cysteine	Cystine
Glutamic Acid	Glutamine	Glycine
Proline	Serine	Tyrosine

Functions of Protein:

Protein plays various very important functions in the body. Most importantly it is responsible for:

- o Growth & Repair of Body Tissue
    - o Muscle tissue – every time you workout you tear down the muscles cells in your body. Protein helps repair, re-build, and

grow your muscle cells after every workout. This is why it's so important to consume a protein source immediately after your workout. It's optimal time to help transform your body for the better.

   o Other body tissues include hair, ligaments, nails, skin, and tendons.

o   Helps Other Bodily Functions

   o Regulates sugar and fat metabolism by balancing the fat storing hormone, insulin.

   o Helps build antibodies to increase your immune system and help fight viruses and infection.

   o Helps blood (hemoglobin) carry oxygen throughout the body. Also transports fat and cholesterol throughout the body.

TYPES of Healthy, Lean Sources of Protein:

High Quality Proteins

   o   High quality proteins contain the 9 essential amino acids in proper proportion. Low quality proteins are missing one or more essential amino acids or contains them in unbalanced amounts. Incomplete proteins are often called "limiting proteins" because they can only build as much tissue as the smallest amount of the necessary amino acid.

   o   High quality proteins have a higher Biological Value (BV). This means your body absorbs high quality proteins more efficiently. The egg is the standard for a high BV for a whole food. It has been given a BV rating of 100%, meaning it contains the most useful and most available protein to be absorbed by the body. Even though other foods may show that they contain more protein than eggs, they may not be as valuable of a source. This is because they may lack the ample amounts of one or more of the essential amino acids.

- For example, on the label, it shows that beans have more protein than eggs. However, the protein in the beans do not have sufficient amounts of all the essential amino acids. This means they are not as valuable in terms of absorbable protein. Therefore, you actually absorb more protein from eggs even though the label says it has less protein per serving.

o You can combine different limiting protein sources to make a full complete protein. This is a process called "complementing proteins". An example of this is combining two limiting proteins like brown rice and beans together. The combination of each food builds an amino acid profile that creates a full complete protein source. A lot of vegetarians employ this strategy.

High Quality Complete Protein Sources	
Protein Source	**Biological Value**
Whey Protein Isolate Powder	110-159
Whey Protein Concentrate Powder	104
Whole Egg	100
Cow's Milk	91
Egg White	88
Cottage Cheese	84
Tuna	83
Fish	82
Beef	80
Chicken	79
Turkey	79
Quinoa	75-82
Casein Protein Powder	77
Soy Protein Powder (I don't recommend)	74

Low Quality Incomplete Protein Sources	
Peanuts	68
Yogurt	68
Oatmeal	58
Rice	57
Whole Wheat	54
Beans	49

Whey Protein Powder

Whey protein powder is now beginning to become more mainstream. It used to be just consumed by bodybuilders and athletes. Fortunately today, everyone from mom and dads to senior citizens are supplementing their diet with whey protein powder. It's a great way to ensure all your meals include a high quality protein source and is quick, easy, and tastes good too. You can add it to your oatmeal in the morning, bake protein bars with it, or add it to your smoothies to make a balanced meal. It's also absorbed very quickly, so it's great to take immediately after your workouts to help repair and grow bigger and stronger muscles.

It is very important for you to stay away from soy protein. No matter what you hear in the media, soy is NOT a health food. If you ever want to awaken the abs within you must avoid soy as it is one of the major causes of stubborn belly fat.

The great majority of soy is genetically modified, contains high concentrations of pesticides, and is also high in phyto estrogenic activity. This means there can be a slight estrogen effect from the protein. You'd be surprised at all the excessive estrogenic compounds found in the modern day food supply. This is bad news for both males and females as overconsumption of soy can cause hormonal imbalances. For men, consuming estrogenic compounds can lead to "man boobs", possible cancer and disease, and excessive accumulation of abdominal fat. For women, estrogenic compounds can throw off the estrogen/testosterone balance which can cause metabolic problems such as excessive belly fat. These same estrogenic compounds are found in pesticides.

Stay away from any food that is soy-based including foods made with soybean oil, beer or anything containing hops, and licorice.

Some foods can actually help fight these estrogenic compounds. These include organic cruciferous veggies such as: broccoli, brussel sprouts, cabbage, cauliflower, leafy greens, garlic, onions, raw honey, teas, citrus fruits, berries, nuts, seeds, avocados, olive oil, fish and krill oil, wild fish, and grass-fed meat and dairy. Do you see a common trend here (hint they're all whole foods)? If you must eat soy, ensure you consume fermented soy products such as tempeh and miso in moderation. Tofu and soy protein are typically not fermented so stay away if you want to get rid of the belly fat.

If you're a vegetarian, try hemp protein, flax protein, alfalfa protein, and rice brown sprouted protein.

Carbohydrates

Discussion of carbohydrates is one of the most controversial topics today in the health industry. The TQT principle applies most to this macronutrient. The effect of carbohydrates on the insulin (fat storing) hormone was discussed in detail earlier. It's pretty scary. That's why you need to be very smart and strategic with your carbohydrate consumption plan. As you now know, eating the wrong carbs, in the wrong quantity, at the wrong times, can wreck havoc on your hormones, creating a fat storing body. This is not what you want.

Carbohydrates should supplement the protein source portion of your meal. Not the other way around. You should never eat a meal or snack that is primarily made of just carbohydrates. Protein is required to regulate the fat storing hormonal effect of carbohydrates.

There are 4 calories in 1 gram of carbohydrate.

Categories of Carbohydrates:

Carbohydrates are split into 2 broad categories according to their structure:

- o Simple Carbohydrates
    - o A simple carbohydrate contains 1 (monosaccharide) or 2 (disaccharide) units of sugar. Therefore, they are broken down into glucose (blood sugar), digested, and absorbed in the blood stream rapidly. Glucose is the body's preferred source of energy.
    - o An example of a monosaccharide is fructose (fruit sugar).
    - o An example of a disaccharide is sucrose.
    - o Food sources of simple sugars include:

- Fruits and fruit juices
- Table sugar or sucrose
- Condiments like jam and honey
- Candy
- Soft Drinks

o Complex Carbohydrates

  o A complex carbohydrate contains more than 2 units of linked sugar. It's known as a polysaccharide. Therefore, they are broken down into glucose (blood sugar), digested, and absorbed in the blood stream SLOWER than simple carbohydrates. This is the category of carbohydrates that the majority of your consumption should come from.

  o Food sources of complex carbohydrates include:
    - Whole grains (bread, oatmeal, rice, pasta)
    - Vegetables (sweet potatoes)
    - Beans and legumes

You can also classify carbohydrates as "starchy" and "green fibrous" carbs.

Examples of starchy carbohydrates include: sweet potatoes, rice, and grains. Essentially these include any carb that contains a lot of starch.

Examples of green fibrous carbohydrates include: green leafy vegetables such as spinach, broccoli, kale, etc.

As mentioned earlier, my clients have dropped the most amounts of excess body fat by eliminating refined sugar and reducing the consumption of grains from their diet. The majority of their daily carbs come from fruits and veggies with a smaller focus on starchy or complex whole grains. These starchy carbs are best consumed earlier in the day when the body requires the slow release of energy and has storage capacity in the muscle and liver glycogen cells.

Functions of Carbohydrates:

The major role of carbohydrates is to provide the body with energy. Glucose is carried in the blood to the muscles, brain, heart and other tissues to be used for energy. The presence of adequate carbohydrates in the body for energy is essential to help decrease the use of protein for energy. Remember, the main function of protein is for muscle building and repairing. Not energy.

As discussed earlier, the spillover effect happens when carbohydrate intake exceeds the body's energy demands and storage capacity in the muscle and liver glycogen. If this happens, the carbohydrates are converted to triglycerides or fat by the liver. They are then stored as fat in different areas throughout the body. BAD!!

TYPES of Healthy Carbohydrate Sources

Glycemic Index:

Carbohydrate-rich foods are ranked from 0-10 according to how fast the sugar gets into the bloodstream. The higher the number, the quicker and more drastic rise in blood sugar occurs after a meal. Foods that raise blood sugar levels quickly are classified as high glycemic carbohydrates. The lower the number, the slower the sugar finds its way into your blood. These foods are classified as Low Glycemic foods.

Try to consume less high glycemic foods or at least combine a small amount of high glycemic foods with lower glycemic foods to get a balance. Always stock your fridge with low glycemic foods. Remember, "Fat-free" doesn't mean calorie free. When food manufacturers remove items from food, in this case fat, they need to add something back in to replace it. More often than not, fat-free means the food manufacturers have added high glycemic ingredients back in.

Another important thing to remember is a term called the glycemic load. Watermelon may have a higher glycemic index but the actual amount of sugar is relatively small because of all the water contained in the watermelon. Therefore it may be less insulin stimulating than lower glycemic ranking foods like corn or bananas, which have higher amounts of carbohydrates.

By adding protein and fat to carbs, you lower the glycemic index of that food. Also eat high protein foods first to start the proper hormonal chemistry. Anything with a lot of fiber will help lower the glycemic index of the food.

For a full list of foods that fall within the low glycemic (best), moderate glycemic (ok), and high glycemic (limit) rankings, visit the official Awaken The Abs Within Website:

http://www.awakentheabswithin.com/glycemic-index-food-rankings/

Kick The "Quick" Sugar Habit

When most people think of sugar they think of cookies, cake, and candy. However, every carbohydrate whether it's fruit, bread, potatoes or pasta turns into sugar in the body. The only difference is how quickly it converts to sugar. Processed foods convert to sugar very quickly because they have been stripped of their fiber, vitamins, germ, and seeds.

Your body is bombarded with sugar every day. Too much sugar is a major cause of obesity and one of the main reasons why your abs are covered with a layer of stored body fat. To much sugar can cause diabetes and also raise your bad cholesterol (LDL) and lower your good cholesterol (HDL).

It's very interesting to compare a typical French diet (high in dietary fat) with a typical North American diet (high in carbohydrates). Studies show the French are significantly less likely to be obese than North Americans. The French diet includes comparable amounts of meat and fish to North Americans but they consume higher amounts of fat and lower amounts of carbohydrates. They only consume approximately 18% as much sugar as North Americans. So why do North Americans consume so much more carbohydrates than the French? One of the reasons is the dietary food guideline set by the North American so-called nutrition experts. They recommend lower dietary fat and higher carbohydrate consumption. The nutrition experts in France promote the opposite. As mentioned earlier, your body has a limited amount of storage space for sugar in the liver and muscle tissues. North Americans are not exercising enough to be able use all the energy being consumed from carbohydrates (sugar). The surplus of sugar that is not burned via exercise is then stored as fat.

Sugar can be described as many different things on food labels. It's sometimes called sucrose (table sugar), dextrose, high fructose corn syrup, as well as many other names. Not all forms of sugar play the same role in our body. Sugar found in natural fruits is in the form of fructose. When you consume a piece of fruit there are natural metabolites to help you digest the sugar. The fiber in the fruit also helps slow down the conversion of sugar in the blood stream. This is a good thing. Fructose is also used as a sweetener in pre-packaged processed foods such as fruit drinks. However the difference is the fiber has been removed. This means the blood sugar levels are raised quickly, which causes havoc on your body. Any food in a can, jar or package more than likely has many different types of unhealthy sweeteners. You need to read food labels. If any sugar appears before the 5th ingredient, it means there is a lot of sugar in the food.

There were studies done with rats that re-affirmed just how addictive sugar is. First, the rats were ingested with cocaine. Then they were given a choice to take more cocaine or sugar. What do you think the rats chose? That's right, the cocaine infused rats chose the intense sweetness of sugar over taking more cocaine.

Try taking a 2-week vacation from consuming refined sugar and I promise you will experience an incredible feeling of health and vitality. Also employ the 5-gram rule. Besides fruits and vegetables, try only eating carbohydrates that contain more than 5 grams of fiber and less than 5 grams of sugar. People need to learn more about the dangers of sugar. It's really a scary thing. It will cut your life short. Once you get scared enough, it can drive you to action. Focus on the benefits of having more energy, losing weight, finding your six pack abs, getting along better with others, having a better libido, and having better focus. Doesn't that sound like enough reason to kick the sugar addiction?

If you are going to have sugar, do not have it alone. Eat a healthy meal first. Before you eat a piece of cake, eat a meal with a balance of protein, unrefined carbs, and healthy fat first. You'll be more satiated and less likely to over due it on the dessert.

Kick the quick sugar habit and begin awakening the abs within!

The Role of Fiber:

Fiber is the part of the food found in carbohydrates that you cannot digest. Fiber rich foods have a high satiety index, meaning they keep you feeling full for longer (helps prevent overeating). You should try to get between 20-35 grams of fiber in your daily diet. Please note, eating more than 50-60 grams of fiber can actually move the food through your system too quickly, meaning the nutrients don't get properly absorbed by the body.

There are 2 categories of fiber:

- Soluble Fiber
    - As the name describes, this fiber dissolves in water. This fiber "traps" waste materials and moves them out of the body. It also slows the absorption of food. Therefore, complex carbohydrates are usually high in soluble fiber and can help slow the release of insulin.
    - It also has been found to lower blood cholesterol levels and potentially help control blood sugar levels.
    - Soluble fiber food sources include:
        - Oats
        - Oatbran
        - Beans and lentils
- Insoluble Fiber
    - Does not dissolve in water. Often referred to as "roughage", it contributes to regular bowel movements.
    - It may be important in the prevention of certain types of cancer.
    - Insoluble fiber food sources include:

- Whole grain breads
- Fruits with edible seeds (strawberries, kiwis, raspberries)
- Broccoli and cauliflower

DIETARY FAT

As discussed earlier, not all dietary fat will make you fat. It's one of the main misconceptions in the health industry. Most people think they need to give up all dietary fat in order to lose body fat. This is not true. Dietary fat plays an important role in keeping you healthy, and in some cases, an important role in fighting fat. Let me say this again, certain fats are essential for proper health and fighting stored body fat.

Fat actually helps control appetite. If you eat a meal comprised mainly of fat and protein you will feel more satiated than when you eat a meal comprised mainly of carbohydrates (both meals containing same number of calories).

The evils associated with dietary fat are related to its excessive use (the "Q" in TQT) and the type of fat being consumed (the first "T" in TQT). When it comes to fat, the first T of the TQT principle is most important. It's consuming the right TYPES of fats and getting rid of the wrong types that will have the most benefit to your abs.

Fat takes up to 4 hours to be completely absorbed in the body. Therefore it also slows the absorption of other nutrients in the body as well. This is especially important to note during post-workout meals. As you know, it is very important to have a quick absorbing protein and carbohydrate source immediately after your workout to flood your muscles with protein and glycogen. By including a fat source in this meal, you are slowing the process. Keep your post-workout meal a low-fat one.

Your body reserves fat as the last resort for energy because glucose is a faster, more efficient energy source. This is why it is often recommended to do morning cardio on an empty stomach (or carbohydrate-less stomach). Since your body has been deprived of all glucose reserves during your overnight fast (sleep), it will turn to stored fat reserves for energy.

There are 9 calories in every gram of fat.

Functions of Dietary Fat:

- Aids in the transport and absorption of micronutrients such as fat-soluble vitamins A, D, E, and K.
- Fat takes a while to digest so it makes you feel full and satisfied at the end of the meal (reduces the risk of overeating).
- Tissue Structure – fat is part of the structural component of all body cells.
- Fat is used in making materials required for metabolic functions and building body tissues.

TYPES of Dietary Fat Sources:

Fat naturally occurs in some foods. In other foods (the ones you are to avoid), it's added in during the processing.

Polyunsaturated Fat:

- These are a healthy fat source that can actually help lower blood cholesterol levels. They are found in:
  - o Nuts & Seeds

- Polyunsaturated fats that contain Omega 3's can help lower blood triglycerides (blood fats). This is why Omega 3's are an ally in fighting excess body fat. Omega 3's are considered Essential Fatty Acids (EFAs) because the body can't produce them on its own. Omega 3's are found in:
  - Salmon, Tuna, Swordfish, Sardines, Trout
  - Flax and Chia Seeds
  - Omega 3 enriched Eggs
  - Krill Oil and Fish Oil

Monounsaturated Fat:

- These are a healthy fat source that can also help lower blood cholesterol. They are found in:
  - Olive oil
  - Nuts & Seeds

Saturated Fat:

- They are found in:
  - Red meat, butter, and dairy such as milk, cheese, and creams
- Coconut Oil
  - Coconut oil is high in saturated fat, however it does not increase blood cholesterol levels. It's a Medium Chain Triglyceride (MCT) form of saturated fat. This MCT fat is strictly used as an energy source and is not stored as body fat. It can also be cooked at high temperatures without burning so it's a highly recommended oil to cook over heat (especially since it's a great source of energy as well).

Trans Fat:

- RED FLAG, RED FLAG, RED FLAG!!
- Trans fats, hydrogenated and partially hydrogenated fats are toxic and unnatural and lead to obesity. They punch holes in cell walls. It's a manufactured form of fat that is used in packaged goods to extend shelf life. Stay away. If you ever want to sabotage your journey to six pack abs, this is the way to do it. It raises blood cholesterol levels and is easily stored as body fat, especially in the abdominal region. They are found in:
    o Most junk food like ice cream, baked goods, cookies, pies, doughnuts, breads, crackers, and chips, soft drinks etc. Essentially anything processed, sugar filled, and considered junk.

Micronutrients

The required micronutrients are classified as:

- Vitamins
- Minerals
- Water

Each micronutrient is essential to maintaining a healthy body. Lets start with Vitamins.

Vitamins

Vitamins are organic substances that are essential in small amounts. Since the body doesn't produce vitamins, they must be obtained from the diet.

12 Types of Vitamins:

The body requires many different vitamins. Each vitamin is unique in structure, metabolic function, and distribution in food. These vitamins are grouped as either:

- **Water-Soluble**
  o Water-soluble vitamins are transported in the body via water. These vitamins are not stored within the body, meaning the body uses what it needs and then excretes the rest out of the body through urine.
  o Since the body doesn't store water-soluble vitamins regular intake is required to prevent deficiencies.
  o Water-soluble vitamins include: Vitamin B1, B2, B3, B5, B6, B12, Folate, Vitamin C

Vitamin	Function	Source
Vitamin B1	Releasing energy from carbohydrates	Whole grains, Seeds, Beans, Nuts
Vitamin B2	Metabolism of fat, protein, carbohydrates and helps remove toxins from liver	Fish, Wheat Germ, Broccoli, Green leafy vegetables

Vitamin B3	Release energy from carbohydrates, metabolism of protein and fat	Poultry, Fish, Meat, Peanuts, Whole Grains, Eggs
Vitamin B5	Glycogen and fatty acid production	Peanuts, Egg Yolks, Fish, Whole Grains, Beans, Nuts
Vitamin B6	Protein and amino acid metabolism	Wheat Germ, Seeds, Chicken, Fish, Eggs, Bananas, Walnuts, Oats
Vitamin B12	Essential function of every cell in the body	Poultry, Fish
Folate	Transporting co-enzymes for metabolism of amino acids	Wheat Germ, Dark Green Leafy Vegetables, Beans, Egg Yolks, Asparagus, Salmon, Whole Wheat
Vitamin C	Antioxidant, tissue repair	Brussel Sprouts, Cranberries, Mango, Kiwi, Sweet Pepper, Broccoli, Strawberries, Tomatoes

- **Fat-Soluble**
    - Fat-soluble vitamins are dissolved in fat and carried throughout the body by chemicals made with fat. These

vitamins are stored in body fat. Over consumption of these vitamins can be toxic.

o Fat-soluble vitamins include: Vitamin A, D, E, and K.

Vitamin	Function	Source
Vitamin A	Vision, healthy skin, bone growth, immunity	Fish Oils, Carrots, Green Leafy Vegetables
Vitamin D	Bone growth, balances mineral levels	Fatty fish, Fish liver oils
Vitamin E	Antioxidant from oxidation damage	Wheat Germ, Olive Oil, Egg Yolk, Almonds, Walnuts, Sunflower Seeds
Vitamin K	Essential for blood clotting	Raw cauliflower, Green leafy vegetables

Minerals

Minerals are inorganic substances that are essential for cell function.

10 Types and Function of the Common Minerals:

Mineral	Function	Source
Calcium	Essential for strong bones, teeth and	Sesame seeds, Yogurt,

	contraction of muscles	Broccoli, Dairy
Magnesium	Essential component of bones, metabolism, and oxidation of glycogen for energy	Whole Grains, Black-eyed Peas, Seeds, Wheat Germ, Dark Green Vegetables, Fish
Phosphorus	Essential for bone formation and vital for ATP	
Sodium	Electrolyte for cellular functions	Beets, Celery, Sea Salt
Chloride	Electrolyte	Sea Salt, Rye, Tomatoes, Lettuce, Celery, Olives
Potassium	Electrolyte, maintains an optimum cellular environment, maintains water balance	Tomato paste, apricots, bananas, pumpkin seeds, almonds, green leafy vegetables, fish
Iron	Central element in the oxygen carrier hemoglobin	Meat, Wheat Germ, Spinach
Selenium	Antioxidant, essential for key enzymes in the body	Tuna, seafood, meat, walnuts, whole grains, vegetables

Chromium	Essential for glucose metabolism, insulin production, and fatty acid and protein metabolism	Whole grains, shell fish, black pepper
Zinc	Essential for metabolism and cell growth	Seafood, pumpkin seeds, sesame seeds, fish, meat, eggs, Wheat Germ

Water

Water is essential for life. More than 60% of the body's weight is water. This makes it the most abundant compound in the body. Humans can exist for several weeks without food but only a few days without water. Drinking enough water can actually cause your body to release the false fat in your system. As mentioned earlier, this false fat is usually in the form of trapped water in the body's tissues. By drinking enough water, you can actually cause this trapped water to release from your system, thus losing this false fat in the meantime. Don't think that by drinking more water, your body will retain more water. Nothing can be further from the truth. When you don't drink enough water you actually produce a water-storing hormone that holds on to the little water you're taking in. Your body is smarter than you think.

Look into a water purification system for your home. Your other appliances (fridge, oven, dishwasher) cost several thousands of dollars and a water purification system is just as valuable. Tap water is about 1 cent/gallon, bottled water $1.50/gallon, reverse osmosis system 20 cents/gallon, acid/alkaline 30 cents/gallon, steam distillation 25 cents/gallon. You must be conscience to try and drink high quality clean water. There can be a lot of impurities in tap water. In many circumstances, there is too much chlorine and chloride in tap water. Adding lemon or lime will also make it more alkaline.

Functions of Water:

Transporter/Detoxifier:

Transports nutrients and oxygen to your cells and carries waste away. Water is key to eliminating toxins from your body.

Temperature Regulator:

Body temperature regulation is dependent on water.

Lubricant:

Water acts as a key lubricant. Without water, your joints would stop moving and seize up.

Your body loses approximately 2.5 litres of water every day through bodily functions such as urination and perspiration. In order to stay hydrated you need to replenish this water. Don't just drink whenever you feel thirsty. When you're thirsty this is the first sign of dehydration. Think of this as a warning sign that you need to drink more water ASAP.

Water Requirements:

The human requirement for water is highly variable. It depends on your activity levels, environment, and current nutrition habits. For example, here are a few factors that increase the requirements for water:

- Physical activity levels
- Live in hot climates
- Low humidity climates
- High altitude area
- Consume high fiber diet
- Consume moderate to high levels of alcohol and/or caffeine

The standard water requirement for an <u>inactive</u> female is 9 cups and 12 cups for <u>inactive</u> males. Since we know you are (or will become) a very active individual with goals to awaken the abs within, you need to be consuming at least half your body weight (in pounds) in ounces of water. For example, if you weigh 200 pounds, you should be drinking at least 100 ounces of water every day. This may seem like a lot, but you will feel so much better once you start drinking more water.

Here are a few strategies to drink more water:

- Always carry a water bottle with you at all times including in your car, in your purse, and at your desk at work.
- Set an alert on your smart phone or in your e-mail program every hour to remind you to drink water.
- Always drink a glass of water before every meal/snack.
- Always choose to drink water rather than soft drinks and fruit juices (except post workout).

- Drink teas (this is a form of water).
- Eat solid foods that contain a lot of water. These include many fruits and vegetables such as lettuce and watermelon.

QUANTITY of Foods

Now that you know the TYPES of foods to eat, it's time to discuss how to calculate the right QUANTITY of each macronutrient. Since the micronutrients come from the foods you eat, by following the TQT principle you will be taking in sufficient amounts of each micronutrient. It is also recommended that you supplement with a multivitamin/mineral as well for your 'micronutrient insurance'. Be aware, all multivitamins are not created the same. There is a lot of crap on the market.

Just because you are looking to burn body fat, it doesn't mean you need or should starve yourself. This will be covered in more detail within the metabolism step. It is crucial to continuously feed your body healthy nutrients every 3 hours to ensure your metabolism and hormones are optimized to burn fat. For most people, this would mean eating 5-6 small meals/snacks per day. This may seem like a lot of food, but it just means you are spreading the SAME AMOUNT of food/calories over more meals. Thus, you're eating smaller meals more frequently.

How many calories should I be eating in a day to awaken my abs (lose the belly fat)?

Your Calorie Calculation:

This is where we're going to set your nutritional numbers…calories, protein, carbohydrate, and fat intake goals.

This is not a one size fits all type question. Everybody is different. Your metabolism is different, your body composition is different, and your activity levels are different.

Here's a simplified calculation to give you a good start in figuring out how many calories you need per day to keep your muscles fed, your metabolism running, and your hormones in balance without overeating.

Lets use John and Jane as examples to show you how to calculate your individual numbers.

John's stats:

- Height = 5'11" (180 cm)
- Weight = 210 lbs (95 kg)
- Age = 30
- Activity level = Works a day job behind a desk and plays recreational hockey 1-2 times per week

Jane's stats:

- Height = 5'3" (160 cm)
- Weight = 150 lbs (68 kg)
- Age = 30
- Activity level = Works a day job behind a desk and walks for 30 mins 1-2 days on the weekend.

Step #1: Find your current total body weight and height

Your total body weight consists of lean body mass & fat mass.

To find your body weight, step on a weight scale and record your number.

To find your height, ask someone to measure you for better accuracy. Stand with your back, feet, glutes, shoulders, and head touching the wall. Use a measuring tape.

John example: 5'11" (180 cm) and weighs 210 lbs (95 kg)

Jane example: 5'3" (160 cm) and weight 150 lbs (68 kg)

For conversion purposes:

- 1 pound (lbs) = 0.45 kilograms (kg)
- 1 inch = 2.54 centimeters (cm)

Step #2: Calculate your Basel Metabolic Rate (BMR)

Your body needs to burn calories just to keep functioning properly. For example, calories are burned to regulate your body temperature, keep your heart beating and your lungs breathing. BMR calculates how many calories you need just for these basic bodily functions. BMR does not represent calories needed for any other activities. BMR essentially represents the calories your body needs to survive if you stayed in bed all day and didn't move.

Lets use the Harris-Benedict equation to calculate BMR:

For men: $(13.75 \times w) + (5 \times h) - (6.76 \times a) + 66$

For women: $(9.56 \times w) + (1.85 \times h) - (4.68 \times a) + 655$

w = weight in kg

h = height in cm

a = age

John example: BMR = *(13.75 x 95) + (5 x 180) – (6.76 x 30) + 66 = 2,069 calories*

Jane example: BMR: *(9.56 x 68) + (1.85 x 160) – (4.68 x 30) + 655 = 1,460 calories*

Remember this does not count calories required for our activity levels (we calculate this in the next step). This is just the calories required to live!

Step #3 Calculate your Activity Factor

Since you move throughout the day, an adjustment to account for your activity levels must be added. This activity level is described by an Activity Factor developed by "McArdle et al 1996".

Activity Factor	Activity Level	Activity Level Definition
1.2	Sedentary	Little or no exercise. Desk job.
1.375	Lightly Active	Light exercise or sports 1-3 days per week.
1.55	Moderately Active	Moderate exercise or sports 3-5 days a week.
1.725	Very Active	Hard exercise or sports 6-7 days a week.
1.9	Extremely Active	Hard daily exercise or sports and physical job.

John example: Activity Factor = 1.375

Jane example: Activity Factor = 1.375

Step #4 Calculate Caloric Needs to <u>MAINTAIN</u> Current Weight

Once you find the activity factor that matches your daily activity level, you would multiple this number by your BMR calculated in the previous step. This calculates how many calories are required to <u>MAINTAIN</u> your current weight (even though you want to lose fat we still need to know this maintenance number).

Maintain Caloric Needs = BMR x Activity Factor

John example: = 2,069 x 1.375 = 2,845 calories

Jane example: = 1,460 x 1.375 = 2,008 calories

Step #5 Calculate Caloric Needs to Lose Fat

Now that you know how many calories are required to maintain your current weight, we need to drop the calories by 500 calories to create a caloric deficit to lose fat.

1 pound of fat equals 3,500 calories. Therefore, to safely lose 1 pound of fat per week you would need to create a caloric deficit by burning 500 more calories than you eat that day. Generally, it's considered safe to lose 1-2 pounds of fat per week.

500 calories per day * 7 days in a week = 3,500 calories

So if John and Jane wanted to safely lose fat, they would set their daily caloric intake to account for a 500-calorie deficit.

John example: 2,845 – 500 = 2,345 calories per day

Jane example: 2,008 – 500 = 1,508 calories per day

Start with a 500-calorie deficit. Don't try to get to ambitious and drop 1,000 calories at the beginning. See how you feel with the 500 deficit and go from there. Remember your body needs energy to function properly and you need energy to workout and build muscle and burn fat. By dropping calories too quickly you can put your body in starvation or hoarding mode where the body holds on to everything and doesn't let it go because it doesn't know if any more food is coming in. That is your body fighting you. You need to work with your body, not against it. Trust the process!

What Should Those Calories Be Comprised Of?

Your Macronutrient Calculation Breakdown:

To effectively burn fat and build muscle you need to be eating protein, carbs, and fat in the proper ratios.

40–40–20 Ratio

The following is a widely used ratio to keep your muscle building hormones and fat burning enzymes working in your favor.

My clients have effectively burned fat and gained muscle using the following 40-40-20 ratio to calculate how their daily calories should be divided:

40% of your daily calories from Lean Protein

40% of your daily calories from Carbohydrates (majority from unrefined low glycemic carbs)

20% of your daily calories from Healthy Fats

To calculate your numbers just follow the calculation example below:

John example: 2,845 – 500 = 2,345 calories per day

Jane example: 2,008 – 500 = 1,508 calories per day

1 gram of protein = 4 calories

1 gram of carbohydrates = 4 calories

1 gram of fat = 9 calories

John's Example Macronutrient Ratio Calculations

Calories:	2,345		
Protein:	40%	938 calories protein/4 calories per gram of protein	938/4 = **235g of protein**
Carbohydrates:	40%	938 calories carbohydrates/4 calories per gram of carbohydrate	938/4 = **235g of carbohydrates**
Fat:	20%	469 calories from fat/9 calories per gram of fat	469/9 = **52g of fat**

Jane's Example Macronutrient Ratio Calculations

Calories:	1,508		
Protein:	40%	603 calories protein/4 calories per gram of protein	603/4 = **151g of protein**
Carbohydrates:	40%	603 calories carbohydrates/4 calories per gram of carbohydrate	603/4 = **151g of carbohydrates**
Fat:	20%	302 calories from fat/9 calories per gram of fat	302/9 = **34g of fat**

Using this simple 40-40-20 ratio shows you how much of each macronutrient should make up your total calorie intake.

Quick Note On No Carb Diets and Extreme Low Fat Diets

People that follow a no carb diet usually experience a quick drop in weight. Initially this drop in weight is coming from lost water (not from lost fat) from the depleted muscle glycogen stores. When you deplete your glycogen stores (by not consuming carbs), you also lose quite a bit of stored water weight. If you cut carbs too much, your energy levels can decline which can lead to a decline in performance at the gym and in life. This is why I always recommend my clients consume the right types of carbs, in the right quantities, at the right times. This gives you the best of both worlds: fat loss and sustainable energy.

By going on an extreme low fat diet, you are limiting consumption of healthy fats that are essential for a properly functioning body and can negatively affect your fat loss efforts, your hormonal processes, and performance. Healthy fat is your friend in fat burning and living a healthy life. In addition to the health benefits of certain dietary fats, most people on extreme low fat diets will often replace the missing calories from fat, with refined carbs full of sugar. Not a good trade off. As mentioned throughout this book, I highly recommend a balanced diet (protein/carbs/fat) comprised of whole/real food.

Does it matter how much of each macronutrient you eat at a time? Yes it matters. For example, Jane may be wondering if she can eat a high carb supper (comprised of let's say 100 grams with little protein) because she didn't have many carbs earlier in the day. This is a no-no. Timing is very important and is the final topic that will be covered in the TQT principle.

TIMING of Foods

Now that you know the correct TYPES of food to eat in the correct QUANTITY, it is now time to learn the correct TIME to eat them. This is the final topic in the TQT principle.

As you now know, different macronutrients cause different hormonal and enzymatic reactions in your body. Therefore, there are specific times when you need to fuel your body with specific macronutrients and other times when your body shouldn't be taking in specific macronutrients.

Protein Intake Timing

It has already been said that protein should be the central building block of your plate. This means protein should be on your plate for all 5-6 meals throughout the day. You need to have protein. Therefore to calculate how much protein you need for each meal, just divide your total daily requirements as calculated in the last section by 5 or 6 (depending on how many meals you're eating). Here's the example:

John's Example Macronutrient Ratio Calculations

Calories:	2,345		
Protein:	40%	938/4 = **235g of protein**	**Divided by 6 meals = 39g per meal**

Jane's Example Macronutrient Ratio Calculations

Calories:	1,508		
Protein:	40%	603/4 = **151g of protein**	**Divided by 6 meals = 25g per meal**

Once again, this means John should try to eat 39 grams of protein during breakfast, mid-morning, lunch, mid-afternoon, supper, and night.

Your body can only absorb so much protein at one sitting. Therefore eating a large protein meal consisting of 100g of protein won't compensate for a missed meal. Always try to consistently eat this set amount of protein at each of your 5-6 meals.

Carbohydrate Intake Timing

This is the important one when it comes to timing. Your body mainly uses carbohydrates (especially starchy carbs) to fulfill its energy requirements. When you've had a few hard workouts, quite a bit of your carbohydrates will turn into muscle glycogen to restore your glycogen levels (this is a good thing and the way nature intended it). If you don't work out and you consume the same amount of carbohydrates, it could be stored as fat since your glycogen levels were not depleted from exercise, thus they'd probably still be at capacity. As described earlier in the The Spillover Effect section of this book, if carb intake grossly exceeds your energy requirements and glycogen storage levels, the carbs can be stored as body fat. This is why you need to consume your carbs (specifically starchy carbs) earlier in the day because this is when your body will use it for energy. At night, the body doesn't need the energy and your glycogen storage levels are likely back at or close to capacity. So by consuming a starchy carbohydrate meal late at night you're giving your body sugar that it has no use for. Thus, it's stored as fat.

We have a limited storage capacity for sugar/carbohydrates. Anything over and above what the body can use (as short term energy or topping up the muscle and liver glycogen) is stored as fat.

Out of your 6 meals, 3 of those meals are comprised of 75% of your daily carbohydrate intake (usually made up of starchy carbs). These meals include breakfast, pre-workout, and post-workout. Regardless of what time of day your workout is, you should always eat a higher carb pre-workout and post-workout meal. You will have sufficient energy requirements and capacity in your glycogen cells to use up this energy without storing it as fat. Your post-workout meal is the one meal where you SHOULD eat simple carbohydrates to quickly spike your insulin hormone to deliver the protein source to the muscles for repair and growth. All other meals should focus on complex carbohydrates as discussed in the section on types of food.

The other 3 meals are comprised of the remaining 25% of your daily carbohydrate intake. Fill out these plates with smaller amounts (if any) of complex carbs and lots of green fibrous vegetables.

John's Example Macronutrient Ratio Calculations

Calories:	2,345		
Carbohydrates:	40%	938/4 = **235g of carbohydrates**	**Breakfast = 20% =** 47g
			Pre-workout (1-2 hours before gym) = **20% = 47g**
			Post-workout (Immediate. No longer than 45 mins after workout) = **35% = 83g**
			Meal #4 = 15% = 35g
			Supper = 10% = 24g
			Meal #6 = 0% = 0g

Jane's Example Macronutrient Ratio Calculations

Calories:	1,508		
Carbohydrates:	40%	603/4 = **151g of** **carbohydrates**	**Breakfast = 20% =** 30g
			Pre-workout (1-2 hours before gym) **=** **20%** = 30g
			Post-workout (Immediate. No longer than 45 mins after workout) **= 35%** = 53g
			Meal #4 = 15% = 23g
			Supper = 10% = 15g
			Meal #6 = 0% = 0g

In this example, John and Jane workout during lunch. This means they have their 3 higher carb meals all earlier in the day. If they worked out after supper, they'd still have a higher carb breakfast plus a higher carbohydrate pre-workout meal (1-2 hours before working out) and the highest carbohydrate meal after their workout (even if that is at 8pm). As mentioned before, your body needs these nutrients at this time, so they will not be stored as fat as long as you put in an intense workout.

Fat Intake Timing

Healthy fats are needed in the body to perform our every day functions. The timing effect of fat consumption mainly has to do around your pre- and post workout meal. Fat slows the absorption of nutrients in the body. Before the workout, fat can make the food digest slower, meaning you may feel like you have a full stomach of food. When working out the body focuses its priority on getting blood to the muscle cells not digesting food that is in your stomach. Therefore, when you eat to soon before a workout, the food just sits in your stomach rather than being properly digested. Most people don't workout at a high level with a full stomach. More importantly, after the workout you want the nutrients to be absorbed as quickly as possible to help re-build and repair your body. Fat slows this process.

You want to consume the majority of your fats during your lower carb meals. The added fat in these meals will also make you feel more satiated even when these meals are low carb.

Lets look at a proper fat intake-timing breakdown based on our example.

John's Example Macronutrient Ratio Calculations

Calories:	2,345		
Fat:	20%	469 calories from fat/9 calories per gram of fat	469/9 = **52g of fat**
			Breakfast = 10% = 5g
			Pre-workout (1-2 hours before gym) = **5%** = 2g
			Post-workout (Immediate. No longer than 45 mins after workout) = **0%** = 0g
			Meal #4 = 30% = 16g
			Supper = 30% = 16g
			Meal #6 = 25% = 13g

Jane's Example Macronutrient Ratio Calculations

Calories:	1,508		
Fat:	20%	302 calories from fat/9 calories per gram of fat	302/9 = **34g of fat**
			Breakfast = 10% = 3g
			Pre-workout (1-2 hours before gym) = **5%** = 2g
			Post-workout (Immediate. No longer than 45 mins after workout) = **0%** = 0g
			Meal #4 = 30% = 10g
			Supper = 30% = 10g
			Meal #6 = 25% = 9g

Similar to the carbohydrate example, John and Jane are working out during lunch. You can customize this to your own situation depending on when your workout times occur.

How Do I Track All This Information To Know If I'm Hitting My Targets?

Keep Track of Your Food Intake with a Meal Planning Software/Journal.

At **http://www.bradgouthrofitness.com/meal-planner-software/** I've created a customizable meal planning software/journal that contains over 200 foods with caloric and macronutrient amounts inputted into the database (protein, carbohydrate, and fat).

By using this software, you will be able to quickly workout precisely what foods you should be eating in the right amounts to maximize your macronutrient intake and ensure you're not taking in excess calories from poor food choices. It will also help you determine when you should be eating and what foods you should eat to hit that meal's macronutrient goals. It keeps an ongoing calculation of your food intake throughout the day so you can see if you're on pace to hit your targets. At the end of the day it shows you the percent of each macronutrient that you hit versus your target. For example, if your protein target was 175 g and it calculated that you took in 165 g, it would show that you accomplished 94% of your day's targeted protein goal.

Another major benefit of the meal planning software is that it keeps you accountable for everything you eat. Since you have to track what you eat, it may make you think twice before consuming that bag of chips.

The meal planning software also contains a tab called Food Items that has approximately 200 healthy foods that can be purchased at any local grocery or health food store. The nutritional breakdowns of the foods are already calculated in the planner.

For a list of all the healthy foods located in the meal planner and the breakdown of calories, protein, carbs, and fat per food 100 grams of that food go to:

http://www.awakentheabswithin.com/macronutrient-breakdown-of-foods/

Even if you don't buy the software, you can still use the list of healthy foods on this website for reference.

Go to: **http://www.bradgouthrofitness.com/meal-planner-software/** to check out the meal planning software.

A Note on Eating Too Much Fruit

People can overdue it on consuming fruit, especially fruit drinks and juices. There is no nutrient in fruit that you can't find in a vegetable. Technically, you never need to eat a fruit (because you can get all the nutrients from vegetables). People can over consume fruit because they are convenient and taste good because of the natural sugar. Males should try not to eat more than 3 small fruits per day and women should try not to eat more than 2 small fruits per day. Most fruit should come from the berry family. For example, bananas are very high in sugar and should only be eaten after strenuous exercise. Vegetarians can tend to over consume fruit. In extreme cases, this can actually lead to diabetes and obesity. For most of history, humans only consumed ½ ounce of fructose from natural fruits per day. Today on average, humans consume over 3 ounces per day. This can play havoc with your metabolic machinery. If you have diabetes in the family or obesity, stay away from dried fruit because it contains too much fructose for the body to process. Don't stop eating fruit. Just don't overdue it.

A Note on Having a "Treat Meal"

Once a week have a treat meal. However, ONLY HAVE A TREAT MEAL when you have successfully followed the plan for all the other week's meals. Go out and celebrate your week of clean eating. You need to have fun along the way to ensure you make this a lifestyle! This treat meal (otherwise called an overfeed) can actually help you lose fat. Yes, I know that sounds crazy, but it's been established that when your body is constantly in a caloric deficit (which is essential to losing fat), your leptin hormone levels drop. A drop in leptin causes a drop in your metabolic rate, higher risk of muscle catabolism, and an increase in your appetite. All of these factors will add up to fat gain. The role of leptin in fat loss will be explained in further detail shortly. However, I wanted to touch on why a treat meal/overfeed is not only good as a reward for a week of nutritious eating, but also can help increase fat loss.

A Note on Alcohol Consumption

Alcohol has a significant effect on your body fat levels. Alcohol calories are higher than protein and carbs. It's about 7g of calories per gram of alcohol. However it's not the calories making people fat. Alcohol makes people fat because it changes the body's chemistry. It causes the body to burn alcohol for energy rather than stored fat for hours after the alcohol was consumed. Put simply, if you're drinking alcohol and binging on bad foods, your body is tied up burning the calories from the alcohol. Thus the calories from the bad food are pretty much stuck in transit and more than likely get stored as body fat.

There are approximately 150 calories in an average serving of beer. However the reason it is more fattening than other alcoholic beverages is because it contains more carbohydrates (which stimulates insulin) and contains hops which are considered a highly estrogenic food. This estrogenic effect could be one of the main causes of all the beer bellies. A glass of red wine contains less calories but the more important thing is you're not stimulating the insulin hormone or the estrogenic effects.

The harder and clearer the liquor such as dry Martinis, vodka, gin, and rum, the fewer the calories and carbohydrates. So if you're concerned about fat gain and have an upcoming party to attend, try sticking with these clear liquor selections but try not to mix with too much soda or juices. Dilute the mix with water if at all possible.

A Note on Fat Burner Supplements

Always consult with your personal physician before taking any fat burner supplement. Fat burners can work by stimulating fat to be released from the fat cells. However you need to exercise to guarantee the body will use that fat as energy. If you decide to take fat burners, make sure you take them before exercise so the fat can make its way to the muscle cells to be burned for energy. A properly formulated fat burner will contain a certain portion of caffeine as caffeine stimulates a brain chemical to release fat from the fat cells. However too much caffeine is not a good thing as it will place too much stress on the body and people can become dependent on it. As mentioned, consult with your physician before trying fat burner supplements.

TQT Conclusion

For best results you should try to hit each macronutrient consumption requirement as closely as possible every day.

Try to not go over the allotted number of calories each day. Remember, to lose fat, you need to create a caloric deficit by moving more and eating less.

Ensure you reach your targets for protein every meal, as this is the macronutrient that is responsible for driving your metabolism.

Be careful not to consume too many starchy carbohydrates such as bread, pasta, and rice. These carb sources have the greatest effect on spiking insulin and cravings for sugar.

Also be sure to adjust your final days meal so that the carbs are coming solely from fibrous, low glycemic vegetables. This will allow for effective fat burning through maximum growth hormone release due to lower insulin levels.

Healthy Balanced Sample Meal Plan

On the following website I've included samples of a healthy and balanced meal plan that is designed to promote fat loss and build muscle.

http://www.awakentheabswithin.com/healthy-balanced-sample-meal-plan/

PLEASE NOTE: this is not a customized meal plan. You will need to figure out your own calorie intake goals (as described earlier) based on your current situation and adjust the food amounts accordingly.

Now that you know how important nutrition is to this new lifestyle, lets take a look at how your metabolism will become one of your best friends during this new journey.

90

SECRET #4:

BOOST YOUR METABOLISM FOR LIFE

What is Metabolism?

Do you really know what metabolism is? The definition of metabolism is the sum total of all the bio chemical reactions that take place in your trillions of cells within a 24 hour day. Put in simpler terms, metabolism refers to the amount of calories your body burns throughout the day to live (i.e. sustain its basic needs). So a faster metabolism means more calories will be burnt, more food can be consumed, and you'll be able to burn excess body fat faster.

Your body has trillions of cells. A large majority of your cells have their own metabolism. Your muscle cells, immune cells, etc. all have their own metabolism. Adenosine Triphosphate (ATP) transfers energy into the cells for metabolism. Having high levels of ATP is considered metabolic success since it's the fuel to allow your metabolism to turn out lots of energy. As a kid you used to produce ATP in abundance. This is what allowed you as a kid to run around forever and eat anything and never gain a pound. Now that you're chronologically older, you may seem to gain fat even after eating one cookie! The reason for this is your body is not as efficient in producing ATP as it was when you were a kid. In other words your metabolism has slowed down. When you're producing lots of ATP, your metabolism is at its peak capacity and is burning greater amounts of fat. Essentially energy creation within the body allows you to burn more stored fat for energy.

There are two sides to metabolism. The first side is called anabolic metabolism. This is the body's ability to rebuild, repair, and replace cells. It is important to remain in an anabolic metabolism state. This creates cellular renewal that leads to creating a more energetic, leaner, and more muscular fat burning body. When you are in an anabolic state you build more lean muscle mass. Since muscle is the metabolic driver, it will help burn and keep off excess body fat. The other side is called catabolic metabolism. This is the body's breakdown of cells including lean muscle tissue. This slows your metabolism and can lead to fat storage.

What Steps Do I Take To Rev Up My Metabolism?

1. Eat Balanced Meals/Snacks Consisting of Thermogenic Foods

Every time you eat, your body uses energy to digest the food. However, there are certain foods that use more energy to digest and process than others. In addition to this, certain foods have a greater influence over the amount calories you burn throughout the day. These thermogenic foods, seasonings, and teas have what we call a high thermogenic value, meaning they can actually make your body burn fat quicker. The most thermogenic source of food is lean protein. The lowest thermogenic source of food are those high in dietary fat. By consuming a diet built around nutrient-dense, natural, lean protein sources, you will help your body burn fat more effectively. Research shows it takes about 30% of the calories from the protein source just to digest and process the food. So if your chicken breast is 100 calories, you're really only storing 70 calories because the body burns the other 30 calories digesting the food.

The following lean protein sources are great thermogenic foods:

- Chicken and Turkey Breast
- Buffalo Bison and other Game Meats (Venison, Elk, etc.)
- Grass Fed Lean Red Meat (Top Round & Sirloin)
- Most Fish and Shellfish
- Egg Whites

I recommend always going with organic and grass fed lean protein sources whenever possible.

Replace the sugary and fattening sauces with the following herbs, spices, and condiments for an even greater thermogenic kick:

- Apple Cider Vinegar (also detoxifies the liver and suppresses hunger levels)
- All Natural Dijon Mustard (improves overall digestion and nutrient utilization)
- White & Red Wine Vinegar (improves blood sugar levels, reduces insulin, and slows digestion)
- Spice it up using these metabolic herbs and spices: Basil, Cayenne, Chili Peppers, Cinnamon, Garlic, Ginger, Hot Sauce, Lemon, Parsley, and Thyme

For most meals and snacks, try to combine a lean protein source with healthy essential fats, lots of green vegetables, and a small amount of unrefined carbs. By doing this, you will create a fat-burning environment within your body.

Here Are A Few Tips To Build A Balanced Fat-Burning Meal:

1. Choose a lean protein source such as one of the items listed above. Season it with cinnamon, cayenne, chili pepper, apple cider vinegar, or hot sauce to really turn up the thermogenic effect.

2. Add lots of green vegetables such as spinach, broccoli, asparagus, etc. Top veggies with a small amount of olive oil (for a healthy fat).

3. For your earlier meals, add a small amount of unrefined carbs such as a sweet potato, brown rice, or oatmeal to give you a slow release of energy throughout the day.

4. Drink green tea after your meal. Green tea contains EGCC (epigallo-catechin gallate), which can help increase your metabolism. Whenever possible (except at night) have a cup of green tea after your meal as it can take 3-4 strong cups to get the necessary amount (270-300 mg) of EGCG. You can also obtain EGCG via green tea extract supplements.

2. Eat Breakfast

We've all heard that breakfast is considered the most important meal of the day. So why is it consistently the most skipped meal?

The term breakfast is a compound of 'break' and 'fast'. Meaning this meal breaks the fasting of food after a long night of sleep. Makes sense doesn't it? Sure it does. And I'm sure you've heard the research that indicates people who skip breakfast are more likely to have less concentration, lack of energy, a lower metabolism, and fat issues. Based on this, it doesn't make sense why some people continuously skip this very important meal!

Why is breakfast so important?

In addition to the reasons already mentioned, consuming breakfast allows the body to refuel its blood glucose (blood sugar) levels after a long night of fasting. Glucose is used as a main source of energy for the body, is essential for the brain, and helps fuel the muscles with energy required for physical activity. Research also indicates that people who eat breakfast tend to eat less calories throughout the day.

But I don't feel like eating breakfast!

I know, I can hear the excuses already..."I don't have time" or "I'm just not hungry in the morning". My answer to those excuses...just do it! Get up 20 minutes earlier by going to bed 20 minutes earlier. Start with eating smaller amounts of food (a piece of fruit) and build your appetite back up to a full serving of breakfast. Or better yet, exercise (even for just 10 minutes) as soon as you get up. You'll definitely be ready to eat breakfast after you finish working out (and waking up) the rest of your body.

What should I eat for breakfast?

If you can't even stand the thought of eating anything in the morning, start small. Grab a small piece of fruit, berries, or a banana and put it in a small bowl of Greek yogurt with a teaspoon of ground flax seed over top.

To add more flavor use a NATURAL SWEETENER like stevia. Always avoid artificial sweeteners like Splenda and Sweet N Low.

You can put this together in less than 3 minutes, it's delicious, and is very light on the stomach. More importantly it is a nutritionally balanced meal since you'll get a source of protein (yogurt), carbs (fruit), and healthy fats (flax seed). As with any new thing, it takes 28 continuous days to become a habit. Once you get your appetite back and your body becomes programmed to crave breakfast (just like supper) you can then add more substance to your breakfast menu.

For example, oatmeal is the staple breakfast meal for most health and fitness experts. In recent years oatmeal has been in the spotlight because of its health benefits. Eating a serving of oatmeal every day can lower cholesterol levels because of its soluble fiber content. The FDA now allows manufacturers of oatmeal to carry a label claiming it may reduce the risk of heart disease in combination with a low-fat diet. As mentioned, it's also a staple in many athletes diet because of the high content of complex carbohydrates (providing a slow release of energy) and water-soluble fiber that slows digestion and stabilizes blood sugar levels.

To make oatmeal a nutritionally balanced meal, add a high quality whey protein isolate powder to the oatmeal after it's cooked and top with berries and walnuts (for a healthy fat).

So if you're not currently eating breakfast, break-the-fast and eat breakfast tomorrow morning!

3. Meal Frequency: Eat Every 3 Hours

In order for your metabolism to operate in peak condition, it requires a constant supply of nutrients such as vitamins, minerals, water, and amino acids. When your body does not receive these nutrients in a timely manner your metabolic rate slows down. It's recommended that you eat smaller meals approximately every 3 hours. This would mean you'd eat 5-6 small meals per day. You may think that is a lot, but it really just means your total caloric intake is spread out over more meals. So you're actually eating the same amount of food but just in smaller quantities at more frequent times. This way you're constantly satiated throughout the day and your blood sugars are balanced. As mentioned earlier, a drop in blood sugar levels is usually the cause of junk food cravings. Eating more frequently also activates leptin. Leptin is actually produced by your body's fat cells. The higher the quantity of active leptin in your body, the more potential your body has for fat burn. To activate leptin, eat more often. As discussed earlier, leptin levels are shown to decline and metabolism slows when meals are skipped or when following a diet that puts you in caloric deficit. This re-enforces the importance of a weekly treat meal/overfeed that is high in carbohydrates (but stay away from anything containing high fructose corn syrup - HFCS). High levels of active leptin can destroy fat cells. Zinc has also been shown to increase active leptin production by 142%. Oysters, wheat germ, and sesame seeds are loaded with zinc. You can also supplement with a multivitamin/mineral to increase your zinc levels.

4. Combine A High Protein Diet With A Resistance Training Program

The combination of eating a high protein diet and participating in resistance training will increase your body's metabolic rate. As mentioned, a high protein meal can increase your metabolic rate by 30%. Compare this to a high carb meal that only increases your metabolic rate by 4%. A high protein diet also increases thermogenic activity. Thermogenesis in the body is like a furnace that creates extra heat by burning excess calories from our fat supplies. The efficiency of your thermogenic system can be the difference between average or high fat storage. How do you add more muscles? **Resistance training!**

Muscles are the number one metabolic factor to our body's ability to burn fat as energy. The majority of fat is shuttled into the engines of the cells within the muscle tissue to be burned for energy. Therefore the amount of muscle you hold on to can determine how your metabolism functions. When you lose muscle, you slow your metabolism. For every pound of fat you lose on a starvation diet, you often take 1 pound of metabolically active muscle tissue with it. Maintaining muscle tissue is the key to a healthy metabolism. Simply put, more muscles = a higher metabolic rate = more fat burn.

5. Is Your Metabolism Feeling Sluggish?

The thyroid plays a major role in how active your metabolism is. A toxic body is one of the biggest causes of a slow thyroid (see Secret #5 on proper detoxification). To support natural thyroid metabolism people should eat more protein and fruits and veggies that are rich in minerals such as iodine, selenium, and potassium. Supplementing with a multi-vitamin can also help people consume these important minerals.

The thyroid produces hormones called thyroxine (T3) and triiodothyronine (T4). T3 is an active hormone in the fat burning process. T4 hormone is non-active but can be converted to the active T3 fat burning hormone. Research has shown the mineral selenium can help in the conversion of non-active T4 to active T3 hormones. Selenium is naturally found in nuts (especially Brazil nuts) and can be supplemented via a multivitamin/mineral.

A slow metabolism may be the result of hypothyroidism. Symptoms can include weight gain, high blood pressure, high cholesterol, and constant fatigue. If you are experiencing these symptoms it is recommended that you see your physician.

So there you have it, by understanding how your metabolism works you can effectively take control of one of the most important factors in the battle against fat storage. A combination of proper exercise, small balanced meal frequency, and a healthy environment (positive thoughts, stress reduction and sleep) all work together to mobilize and burn the stored body fat within your body. As mentioned above, detoxing the body of toxins can help increase the thyroid. Lets discuss this further now.

SECRET #5:

DETOX YOUR BODY FOR FAT LOSS

An often over looked area of fat loss is the role of detoxification within the body (specifically the liver). Simply keeping your liver clean can help you lose fat much easier.

What causes a toxic liver? Many things can cause toxicity of the liver. These include:

- Food
    - o Specifically unnatural, processed, and chemical laden foods. i.e. junk food filled with sugar and unnatural chemicals
- Drinks
    - o Excessive alcohol consumption
    - o Soft drinks and sugar loaded "Fruit Drinks"

- Skin Products filled with unnatural chemicals
    - Anything you put on your skin such as:
        - Soap
        - Shampoo & Conditioner
        - Deodorant
        - Sun block
- Environment
    - Pollutants in the air (smog and second hand cigarette smoke)
- Too many unnatural medications

All of these causes can lead to a toxic liver. When your liver is in a toxic state you create nasty metabolites that the liver can't breakdown. This causes all these toxins to be thrown into your bile. The role of bile is to metabolize fat. Unfortunately when the toxins are thrown into the bile, the bile thickens, causing problems for the body to break down the fat in your system (drinking pure Lemon Water can help thin out the bile – more on this in a bit). Ultimately, if your body can't break down the fat, your body will store it, thus hindering your potential for a lean sexy flat stomach.

Regardless of how clean you eat, or how safe you are with the skin products you use, the toxins in the environment are hard to escape. Therefore it is important for everyone to implement detox methods into your health regiment.

Drinking specific liquids (see examples below) can help get all the junk (fatty globules) out of your lymphatic system.

Here are a few ways to help detoxify your body:

1. Lemon Water

One of the best daily practices you can follow to help detox your body is to drink a glass of freshly squeezed lemon water first thing in the morning (on an empty stomach).

If you'd like a simple and inexpensive way to improve the way you look and feel, implement this practice into your everyday routine. You may be thinking…but I always drink coffee as soon as I get up. This doesn't mean you can't drink coffee. It just means you should postpone that cup of coffee for 30 minutes until your body digests the lemon water.

Here's how to implement drinking Lemon Water as a daily practice first thing in the morning:

1. Wake up.

2. Go straight to the kitchen and pour a glass of room temperature water (if you have digestive problems, use hot water).

3. Cut a lemon in half (don't use bottled lemon juice as it can contain sulphites which many people are allergic to).

4. Squeeze the juice of the lemon directly into the glass of water. Water should turn cloudy.

5. Drink.

6. Repeat the next morning.

It's that simple. But why should you do this?

Health Benefits of Lemon Water

- **Great for Fat Loss:** lemon water can help burn fat faster. When the liver is full of toxins it can't metabolize fats as efficiently. The toxins thicken the bile, which eliminates its ability to metabolize the fat. Lemon water helps thin out the bile thus increase fat mobilization.

- **Helps Liver Eliminate Toxins and Waste Products:** the liver has various roles in the body including detoxification, protein synthesis, and production of bio chemicals to aid in proper digestion. Lemon water increases the livers detoxifying enzymes and helps the liver carry out these functions more efficiently.

- **Lemon Water is Alkalizing:** the body functions best in a more alkaline state and cancer cells tend to breed in an acidic body. Unfortunately due to the foods most people eat, the things they expose their skin to, and the environment they live in, most people's bodies are very acidic. Lemons are very alkalizing to the body and blood.

- **Rich Source of Vitamins and Mineral**s: contains vitamin C (anti-oxidant & helps immune system), vitamin B (energy production), riboflavin (tissue repair, growth, & development) and minerals like calcium, phosphorus, and magnesium (these minerals all help build strong bones & teeth).

- **Terrific for Skin Care:** Lemon water can act as an anti-aging remedy by removing wrinkles and improve the overall appearance of your skin. Your skin can't look healthy if your body is holding onto toxins.

2. Other Detoxifying Drinks

- Powdered cleansing Green Drinks containing:
    - o Phytonutrients, probiotics, and antioxidants

- Tea
    - o Green tea
    - o Matcha tea
    - o Herbal tea
- Cranberry water (homemade unsweetened)
    - o Purchase unsweetened 100% pure cranberry juice.
    - o If you purchase the right type of pure/natural unsweetened cranberry juice, it's very potent. Ensure you dilute it with water. Proper ratio is a 4-part water to 1-part cranberry juice. Cranberry Water helps open up the livers detox pathways.
- Water
    - o Drink at least half your weight (in pounds) in ounces. For example, if you weight 200 pounds, drink at least 100 ounces of water everyday to help flush the toxins out of the system.

3. Consume lots of Veggies

- Veggies contain loads of antioxidants that can help your body metabolize the toxins in your body. Consuming one antioxidant in particular, Glutathione, will surely help your body rid itself of toxins. This antioxidant is found naturally in veggies such as kale and brussel sprouts. Also focus on adding more broccoli, beets, cauliflower, red cabbage, and arugula to your plate.

You now understand the importance of detoxing your body for fat loss. Now all these secrets to lose belly fat may sound good, but do you belief you can do it? If you don't, you've already lost the game. Read the next secret regarding the power of belief. If you believe, you can achieve!

SECRET #6:

THE POWER OF BELIEF – THE MENTAL AND RELATIONSHIP ASPECT OF FAT LOSS

Physiology and psychology are closely linked. The health of your body is often dependent on the health of your mind. Exercise is one component of fat loss. Diet is another. But most people forget about the mental and relationship aspect of fat loss. It's your belief and thoughts that will essentially lead to your actions. Over 50% of people that begin to exercise quit within the first 6 months. Is this because they do not have self-belief? How you think will determine how well you do with exercise. If you think you can't accomplish your goals, you've already failed. Act as if it is impossible for you to fail with your exercise routine. Positive belief patterns are what successful people strive on. You must change how you perceive yourself and live a life of abundance. You have the power through belief to do things you never thought were possible as long as you give up the belief that you can't have it.

To change your destiny, you first have to change your perceptions. Believe you can lose the excess belly fat and awaken the abs within!

There is always someone in worse shape than you that has accomplished results that you may think are impossible. That person isn't more special than you. They don't have special powers. The only thing they had is a strong self-belief that they could do it! You have everything within you to make this work. You just need the right education and actionable steps to set you in the right direction. You now have that with this book.

Research shows that people that have positive self-belief are much more likely to stick to exercise plans and accomplish their goals than people with negative self-confidence who feel they can't do it. If you have a positive feeling towards exercise, you will want to exercise more. It all starts in your head. If you think you can, you can!

Keep it positive and keep your eye on the end goal. Find a few inspirational photos of people and put it on the fridge. Every time you go to the fridge to cheat, you'll see the inspirational pictures and they'll bring you back on track.

Also be sure to break down your end goal into smaller, achievable milestones. And most important of all, celebrate your successes. This is not going to be easy. To keep yourself motivated, always find ways to reward yourself (in a healthy way).

Statistics show that 1/3 of women at any given time can be shown to be starting or finishing a diet. So obviously if diets worked they wouldn't be moving on to another diet. Remember, this is a lifestyle!

Everyone is looking for the quick fix. People want the greatest results in the least amount of time. You need to realize that this is a lifestyle change not a quick fix. You have to believe in yourself and make the necessary changes. Don't put it off for another day.

Break the pattern of negative thinking. Try this exercise. Put an elastic band on your wrist and snap it every time you think a negative thought. You will quickly realize how many negative thoughts you think in a day. Being aware of this will help you to stop the negative thought and replace it with a positive one.

For example, if negative thoughts about the gym enter your mind because you think you don't have the energy to go…stop the thought immediately and re-phrase it so that you say to yourself, "if I go to the gym I'll feel great about myself because of the natural high that exercising produces in the body".

Words have so much power. The words you say and think describe your world and can create it. It's believed that your self-talk creates 100% of your results. To accomplish your goals you need to learn how to filter out all the negative talk. This is the talk that includes, "I can't do it", "I'll never get the body I want", etc. Only use positive self-talk. The right words at the right times can give you the boost you need to accomplish your goals. The words you use to describe yourself can become your habits, which then become your destiny. You need to feel like you've already accomplished your goals. Act as if you've already lost the fat.

Try not to use negative damaging words such as worry, hard, difficult, bad, and hate. Are your words helping you achieve your goals or are they holding you back?

Stress

Stress is only produced if you interpret an event or action in a negative way. Perception equals reality. You can control how you react to these situations. It's all about putting it into perception. At the end of the day, is it really that big of a deal? Will you still have a family? Is anyone going to die because of it? More than likely in a couple weeks you won't even remember that this event occurred.

Stress actually creates an environment that makes people fat. When you worry about things you create a stress response that releases cortisol. As discussed earlier, cortisol strips the muscle of nitrogen which leads to losing muscle mass. This can ruin and lower your metabolism every time you worry. Worse yet, most of these receptors for cortisol are found in the abdominals. This leads to an increase in abdominal fat even if the person is very thin.

So to make this clear, stress causes:

1.   More fat to be stored in the abdominal region
2.   Muscle to be stripped which slows down metabolism
3.   The killing of brain cells that produce feel good chemicals such as dopamine and serotonin. When your brain is low on these chemicals it can lead to food cravings that will add more fat!

Laugh, Smile, Exercise, and Sleep More

Laughter builds up the immune system and reduces stress levels. Smiling also helps reduce stress. In a study with women with botox, it was found they were actually happier because the botex physically made them smile more.

Exercise such as resistance training and cardio actually helps burn off tension, stress, and anger. It does wonderful things for the body and the brain since they are all connected.

Sleep researchers state that over half the American population is sleep deprived. If you're interested in losing body fat and gaining muscle then sleep is no longer an option. Consistent quality sleep is a necessity. You should be spending 1/3 of your life sleeping. This will dictate how healthy the other 2/3's of your life is. Based on most research, 7-8 hours of sleep is required for optimal health. There are a few outliers that may require less but they are not the majority.

Your body is designed to expect 7-8 hours of sleep. Sleep is the greatest asset you have to rebuild, replace and repair your bodies worn out cells. It also allows your body to maintain an effective immune system and burn body fat. Sleep is a time when your metabolism switches from the catabolic (breakdown) to an anabolic metabolism (rebuilding). During sleep the human growth hormone is produced in its highest amount. Human growth hormone helps your body to stay healthy, young, and assists in keeping the body fat off.

A good night's sleep also helps manage stress. As you know, in times of stress the body produces a hormone called cortisol. This hormone strips the body of lean muscle tissue (i.e. the metabolic driver). Get more sleep and stress less.

You need to prepare yourself for sleep. Get into a sleep routine. Research shows that people who are exposed to too much light before bed have decreased production levels of the sleep hormone melatonin. Ensure your room is dark with no access to TV or computers. This means get the TV out of your bedroom and don't bring the laptop to bed. The last 30 minutes before you go to bed should be considered your relaxing time. Don't drink alcohol, coffee or other stimulants during this time. Also try not to watch the news or violent television programs. Try taking a soothing bath with candles, listening to relaxing music, or meditation. It's all about finding things to turn off your brain to prepare for a relaxing and deeper sleep.

Tryptophan is an amino acid that can make you feel sleepy. It is responsible for manufacturing the feel good brain chemical serotonin. Serotonin then converts to the sleep hormone melatonin when in darkness. Unfortunately tryptophan is the least common denominator in most protein containing food and is easily degraded when stressed. A protein shake with high levels of tryptophan can help you go into a deeper and more restorative sleep.

How do your personal relationships affect your body fat levels?

Did you know statistics show that people in love tend to be in better physical health? When you're happy and in love, you can experience a natural high on a brain chemical called dopamine. This high can lead you to eat less, sleep better, and lower your overall stress levels within the body. These are all positive steps that can lead to lower body fat levels.

Although this isn't a relationship book, it does make sense to quickly touch on the importance of positive relationships in the overall health picture. Relationships take effort. So continuously work and grow together with your loved ones. Take the time to learn the love skills. Trust one another. Grow your emotional intelligence (especially you guys). And finally take responsibility and keep the communication channels open.

Lets move on to the last secret. Exercise!

SECRET #7:

DESIGNING A FAT BURNING EXERCISE PLAN

At this time I hope you've realized how important all the OTHER secrets are in awakening the abs within. In fact they are more important than the physical act of exercising, I can't stress this enough, nutrition is the main factor in shedding the extra layer of body fat from your abs. This is why such a large percentage of this book is spent discussing nutrition.

However, now is the time to cover what you should be doing in the gym. And guess what…it's not about spending hours on the treadmill and doing thousands of crunches! The 7th and final secret covers cardio, direct training of the abs, and most importantly, full body resistance training. That's right, following a properly designed, full body resistance-training program will elicit the most beneficial fat burning and muscle building hormonal response. Before we get into it, lets set the record straight…

Priorities

Do you think you don't have time to exercise? MAKE TIME. There's always time to exercise. If you're watching TV, do your exercises during the commercials, march on the spot when you're talking on the phone, or contract your abs while driving (it's called the vacuum). There's always someone busier than you that is finding the time to exercise.

Research shows 3 sets of 10 minutes of walking at different times of the day is just as effective in burning body fat and calories as 30 minutes of straight walking. Stop making excuses and start taking action. It's all about choices. Make the right ones by starting now.

This is your life we're talking about. Make exercise a priority.

Lets get into it...

The Perfect Fat Burning Workout Program

This fat burning workout program consists of a warm-up, a resistance training program for both beginners and more advanced lifters, cardio programs, direct abdominal training, and stretching.

Always ensure you properly warm up before any kind of workout. This will help increase your performance and reduce risk of injury.

If you are just beginning to workout, I highly recommend you start with the beginner program. This can be done at home (if you don't have a gym membership) or at the gym. Complete this workout first and then move on to the more advanced program once you feel comfortable lifting heavier weights.

The more advanced lifting program is comprised of full body workouts that combine upper and lower body multi-joint compound exercises.

Once you complete the weight lifting portion of the workout, you can then complete 10-15 minutes of direct ab training as outlined in the following program.

To round out your exercise program, I recommend completing the indicated cardio programs on your off lifting days.

Warm Up

Before you begin any workout, always ensure you go through a proper warm up. Ensure you never work a cold muscle. Your warm up should consist of 5-10 minutes of light training on the treadmill, bike, elliptical, rower, etc. You could also complete 5-10 minutes of dynamic stretching (not static stretching) using continuous movement to warm up the cold muscle. Arm circles, body weight lunges, and leg swings are all examples of dynamic stretches. Static stretching should be completed post-workout. Static stretching is simply a stretch where the end position is held for 30-60 seconds. You should not complete static stretching on cold muscles as it can increase the risk of injury.

Warm up Benefits:

- Gets the blood flowing and properly warms up the working muscle.
    - o By warming up, the blood vessels dilate to increase blood flow, which lowers stress on the heart.

o Overall performance, including speed and strength are enhanced in warm muscles as a warm muscle can contract more forcefully and relax quicker.

o The risk of injury by over stretching, straining, or pulling a warm muscle is far less than injuring a cold muscle. This is because a warmed muscle has greater elasticity. Also the range of motion around the joints become greater and reduces the risk of muscle stiffness.

- Mental Focus

    o Most people have a lot going on in their lives. When you're in the gym, your mind needs to be focused on the task at hand. You can cause severe injuries when your mind is elsewhere when you're lifting heavy weights. Take time during the warm up to not only prepare your muscles but also prepare your mind to focus on having a great workout.

Cardio

Cardio (aerobic) training is a great way to enhance the fat burning process as long as it is used in combination with a proper resistance-training program. Unfortunately, people rely too much on cardio training as their only source of burning fat. As discussed earlier, excessive cardio without proper resistance-training can catabolize (breakdown) your lean muscle tissues thus reducing muscle mass (the metabolic driver of the body) and slowing your metabolism. Ensure your workout program does not just consist of 100% cardio.

Types of Cardio Programs

There are numerous variations of cardio that can be used to help burn excess body fat. Some are more effective and efficient than others. As with all exercise, if you continuously do the same cardio routine over and over again your body will adapt to its environment and become more efficient at using less energy for what was once a struggle. Alternating high intensity with low intensity cardio programs will keep the body from adapting as quickly, meaning it will require more energy to do the job. This is ideal when you want to be using stored fat for energy. Always keep your body guessing by switching between these cardio programs. Here is a breakdown of a few options that are most beneficial to burning body fat:

High Intensity Interval Training (HIIT)

HIIT require strong bursts of aerobic exercise where your heart rate approaches 70-80% of its maximum heart rate (MHR) for a brief period of time (interval). After the high intensity interval is completed, you reduce the intensity to allow your heart rate to drop back to 50-60% of MHR.

To calculate your max heart rate use the following formula:

MHR = 220 – Age

For example, if you were 30 years old your MHR would be calculated as follows:

Max Heart Rate = 220 – 30 = 190 Beats Per Minute (BPM)

To calculate the high intensity interval portion (80% of your MHR) use the following formula:

MHR x 80%

High intensity interval portion = 190 x .80 = 152 Beats Per Minute

To calculate the low intensity interval portion (60% of your MHR) use the following formula:

MHR x 60%

Low intensity interval portion = 190 x .60 = 114 Beats Per Minute

Therefore for the high intensity interval portion of the cardio training you need to increase the intensity. This can be done by increasing the speed, incline, etc. until you're maintaining a heart rate around 152 BPM for the allotted interval period. You should be winded and have a hard time carrying a conversation during this interval. Once the interval is completed you would decrease the speed, incline, etc. to allow your heart rate to drop to 114 BPM. Once the interval is completed you go back to the high intensity interval and repeat for a specified amount of intervals. The higher your cardio fitness level the quicker your HR will drop during recovery intervals. This is a great way to measure your cardio improvement progress as you continue with this training. For example, for your first few HIIT cardio sessions, it may take you 3 minutes to bring your HR back down to 60% of MHR. As you progress and increase your cardio fitness levels it will eventually take you 2 minutes to properly recover and then 1 minute.

Most cardio equipment has a heart rate monitor built in to the handgrips. If your equipment does not include this built in feature you can buy a HR monitor watch. This watch will show you exactly where your heart rate is so you can properly stay within the proper HR zone and increase/decrease intensity as needed.

HIIT interval training is a more advanced cardio program but highly effective and efficient.

Example of an intermediate HIIT Program

1. 20 x 60 second intervals (10 high intensity & 10 low intensity intervals). For a total of 20 minutes.

2. Each interval consists of 60 seconds of high intensity (80% of HRM) followed by 60 seconds of recovery (or however long it takes to bring you back to 60% of HRM)

3. In addition to the 20 minutes of intervals, complete 3 minutes of warm up increasing the intensity within the 3 minutes until you reach 70% of MHR.

4. Once you complete the 3 minute warm up (hopefully you're at 70% of MHR but it's not mandatory) you should increase to the high intensity interval during the 4th minute. Aim to keep your effort up for the full 60 seconds and pay attention to where your HR goes. You want to get it to 80%. If you go past it, drop the intensity until

you find your sweet spot.

5. Once the 60 seconds is up, drop the intensity during your recovery interval. Watch your HR as you want it to drop to 60% of MHR. Don't go back into the high intensity interval until your HR drops.

6. Repeat until you complete 10 intervals of high and low intensity.

7. Once finished, allow for a 3 minute cool down, ensuring your HR drops below your 60% MHR.

You can use the bike, rowing machine, elliptical, stair climber, jump rope, etc. Any form of exercise that increases your HR and maintains it during the timed interval.

For a beginner HIIT routine, start out with 5 high intensity intervals and work your way up to completing 10 high intensity intervals. For a more advanced HIIT routine, decrease the work-rest ratio by completing 10 x 60 seconds high intensity intervals followed by a 30 second rest ratio. Only move onto more advanced programs when your HR falls quick enough during the rest ratio.

Sprints

Sprints are a more advanced level of HIIT but one of the most effective. If you're in good enough shape, you should try incorporating more sprinting into your cardio routines.

Here are two examples of sprinting cardio programs:

Intermediate/Advanced Sprinting Cardio Program

Sprint #1 – 50 yards

Rest #1 - 30 second rest

Sprint #2 – 50 yards

Rest #2 – 30 second rest

Sprint #3 – 50 yards

Rest #3 - 30 second rest

Sprint #4 – 50 yards

Rest #4 - 30 second rest

Sprint #5 – 75 yards

Rest #5 - 60 second rest

Sprint #6 – 75 yards

Rest #6 - 60 second rest

Sprint #7 – 75 yards

Rest #7 - 60 second rest

Sprint #8 – 75 yards

Rest #8 - 60 second rest

Sprint #9 – 100 yards

Rest #9 – 90 second rest

Sprint #10 – 100 yards

Rest #10 – 90 second rest

Sprint #11 – 100 yards

Rest #11 – 90 second rest

Sprint #12 – 100 yards

Rest #12 – 90 second rest

Advanced Hill Sprinting Cardio Program

Hill Sprint #1 – 20 yards

Rest #1 – time it takes to walk back down the hill

Hill Sprint #2 – 20 yards

Rest #2 – time it takes to walk back down the hill

Hill Sprint #3 – 20 yards

Rest #3 – time it takes to walk back down the hill

Hill Sprint #4 – 20 yards

Rest #4 – time it takes to walk back down the hill

Hill Sprint #5 – 20 yards

Rest #5 – time it takes to walk back down the hill

Hill Sprint #6 – 30 yards

Rest #6 – time it takes to walk back down the hill

Hill Sprint #7 – 30 yards

Rest #7 – time it takes to walk back down the hill

Hill Sprint #8 – 30 yards

Rest #8 – time it takes to walk back down the hill

Hill Sprint #9 – 30 yards

Rest #9 – time it takes to walk back down the hill

Hill Sprint #10 – 30 yards

Rest #10 – time it takes to walk back down the hill

Steady Pace

Steady state cardio is a form of lower intensity cardio that keeps your heart rate in a consistent zone for a longer time. The speed is normally maintained at a faster than normal walking speed on a steep incline (without holding on to the bar if you're on a treadmill). You should still be able to carry a conversation while training in this intensity. Since this is a lower intensity program you should do this for longer periods of time.

Example of a Steady State Cardio Program:

1. Start on a machine with a low effort setting and slowly increase the intensity over the next 3 minutes until you reach 70% of your MHR. You can increase the intensity by increasing the speed, resistance, or elevation of the machine.

2. Make a note of the speed, resistance, elevation of the machine that takes you to 70% of your MHR. Within a few weeks as you progress, you will notice you will need more speed, resistance, elevation to bring you up to 70% MHR.

3. The goal is now to maintain this level for the full 60 minutes, forcing the body to supply a steady stream of energy that is above what is normally required.

4. A cool down is required after your program. Allow your HR to come down to 50% MHR and then you're finished.

All cardio machines such as treadmill, stepper, rower, bike, elliptical, etc. are ideal for steady state cardio.

If you find 60 minutes on one machine is too much for your boredom, you can switch to another machine and bring the intensity back in line with the previous machine.

When Do I Complete My Cardio Routine?

There are many different strategies for completing cardio at different times during the day. It really depends on what your schedule will allow. Here are a few options:

Option #1 Early morning cardio

Many people realize the greatest fat burning benefits of cardio early in the morning. This is because cardio first thing in the morning can spike your metabolism for many hours after you are out of the gym thus burning more calories throughout the day. If you can make the time, you could follow this morning cardio routine with a resistance training routine in the evening.

Option #2 Resistance Training + Cardio Session

If you don't have the time to complete two workout routines in a day, you could combine your resistance training program with your cardio program during the same session. Always complete the resistance training program first, followed by the cardio program. The rationale for this is simple. Research has shown that, depending on your fitness level; it can take approximately 20 minutes for your body to begin burning fat for energy. During these 20 minutes you're essentially burning sugar (carbohydrates). Your body is like a car. It takes a while to warm up. Your body uses this warm up to prepare the body to release the fatty acids to be burned for energy. It doesn't happen instantly. Therefore, if you stay on the treadmill for 25 minutes you could have only been burning fat for energy for 5 minutes. On top of this, you've depleted your energy before you begin your resistance training portion of the workout causing you to not be able to lift as heavy or intense as you could of if you didn't do cardio first. Lets look at this scenario in reverse. By completing your resistance training first, not only do you have the required energy to lift heavy and hard, you also have properly warmed up your body enough so that when you begin cardio, the fatty acids are released and ready to be burned for energy immediately.

Option #3 Cardio Training Off Day

The third option is to complete your cardio training on your resistance training off days. For example, if you complete resistance training on day 1, 3, and 5; you would complete your cardio on days 2 and 4.

As mentioned above, it really all depends on how much time you can devote to your health. I personally have tried all three options but have experienced the greatest results using option #1. By spiking your metabolism early in the morning you can actually feel the body burning excess body fat. All bodies react differently to different stimuli. Give each option a try and see which works best for you.

Everyone's recovery time is different, however most people respond best with 3-4 lifting sessions and 2-3 cardio session per week.

This allows you to lift weights every other day (giving your muscles 48 hours rest), cardio on off-lifting days, and then 1-2 complete days off.

Follow this frequency and you shouldn't be in any risk of over training or not stimulating the body enough.

How Long Should My Sessions Be?

Keep sessions between 45 and 75 minutes. If you're working out hard enough you shouldn't be able to continue past 75 minutes. There are also numerous studies that show prolonged workouts can increase the level of cortisol production. As you've read earlier, you do not want cortisol to be wrecking havoc on your hard earned muscle.

Exercise Database

All the exercises listed below are "Awaken The Abs Within" approved exercises. Focus on adding these to your workouts to ensure you're creating a metabolic and fat burning hormonal environment in your body.

For picture demonstrations with instructions of these exercises visit:

http://www.awakentheabswithin.com/awaken-the-abs-within-exercises/

Jumping Jacks

Jump to a position with the legs spread wide and the hands touching overhead and then return to a position with the feet together and the arms at the sides. That's one rep.

High Knees

Stand with both feet together. Start running in place getting your knees as high as possible. Once you raise both knees once, that's one rep.

Dumbbell Squat and Press

Begin with your back straight, feet shoulder-width apart and dumbbells at shoulder height. Lower yourself by pushing your hips back until you reach about 90 degrees of flexion in the knees. Keep your mid-section tight and look straight ahead. Rise up out of the squat with a slight explosion and simultaneously press the dumbbells overhead. End the movement by lowering the dumbbells back to shoulder height. That's one rep.

Push Up

Lay chest-down, hands at shoulder level, palms flat on the floor and slightly more than shoulder-width apart, and your feet together and parallel to each other. Straighten your arms as you push your body up off the floor. Pause for a moment. Lower your body slowly towards the floor. That's one rep.

Lunges

Lunge forward with first leg. Land on heel then forefoot. Lower body until knee of rear leg is almost in contact with floor. Return to original standing position. Repeat by alternating lunge with opposite leg. That's one rep.

Chair Dips

Place your hands on a chair or bench. Keep your elbows close to your body. Slowly lower your body downward. Then extend your arms, raising your body upward and supporting your weight with your arms. That's one rep.

Mountain Climber

Place hands on floor, slightly wider than shoulder width. While holding upper body in place, alternate leg positions by pushing hips up while immediately extending forward leg back and pulling rear leg forward under body, landing on both forefeet simultaneously. Once you bring in both knees, that's one rep.

Mountain Climber on Swiss Ball

Place hands on swiss ball. While holding upper body in place, alternate leg positions by pushing hips up while immediately extending forward leg back and pulling rear leg forward under body, landing on both forefeet simultaneously. Once you bring in both knees, that's one rep.

Burpee

Begin in a squat position with hands on the floor in front of you. Kick your feet back to a pushup position. Immediately return your feet to the squat position. Leap up as high as possible from the squat position. That's one rep.

Dumbbell Renegade Row

Start in a push up position, gripping a pair of dumbbells. Pull one dumbbell up to your arm pit. Then repeat with the other arm. That's one rep.

Kettlebell Swing

Straddle kettlebell with feet slightly wider apart than shoulder width. Squat down with arms extended downward between legs and grasp kettlebell handle with both hands with an overhand grip. Position shoulder over kettlebell with taut low back and trunk close to vertical. Pull kettlebell up off floor, slightly forward, just above height of ankles. Immediately dip down slightly and swing kettlebell back under hips. Quickly swing kettlebell up by raising upper body upright and extending legs. Continue to swing kettlebell back down between legs and up higher on each swing until height just above head can be mantained. Swing kettlebell back down between legs. That's one rep.

For the One-Arm Dynamic Kettlebell Swing, use the same form however just use one arm and dynamically let go of the weight at the top of the motion and quickly grab it with your other arm while it's in the air.

Plank

Lie facedown on a mat. Place forearms on mat, elbows under shoulders. Place legs together with forefeet on floor. Raise body upward by straightening body in straight line. Hold.

Side Plank

Lie on your side on a mat. Place forearm on mat under shoulder perpendicular to body. Place upper leg directly on top of lower leg and straighten knees and hips. Raise body upward by straightening waist so body is ridged. Hold. Repeat with opposite side.

Jump Rope

Using a jump rope, grasp handles with both hands and rotate rope overhead and repeatedly jump for desired time or jumps.

One Legged Dumbbell Squat

Stand with dumbbells grasped to sides. Balance on one leg with opposite leg extended straight leg forward as high as possible. Squat down as far as possible while keeping leg elevated off of floor. Keep back straight and supporting knee pointed same direction as foot supporting. Raise body back up to original position until knee and hip of supporting leg is straight. Return. That's one rep.

Dumbbell Renegade Row + Side Plank

Start in a push up position, gripping a pair of dumbbells. Pull one dumbbell up to your arm pit then continue to raise arm upward by straightening waist so body is ridged and arm is directly over shoulder. Pause and repeat with other side. That's one rep.

Lying Hip Raise

While lying flat on the floor (hands can be under your glutes) raise legs up so there is a 90 degree angle formed at the hips (this is starting position). Thrust hips up in the air with legs reducing the angle between hips and shoulders. That's one rep.

V-Ups

Lay down on floor with hands overhead. Simultaneously raise straight legs and torso. Reach toward raised feet. Return to starting position. That's one rep.

Inverted Row

Lay on back under fixed horizontal bar. Grasp bar with wide overhand grip. Keeping body straight, pull body up to bar. Return until arms are extended. That's one rep.

Ab Wheel

Begin by kneeling on the floor, and hold both sides of the wheel. Roll the wheel forward, and lower your body as far as you can without arching your back. Then, use your abs to pull yourself back to the starting position. That's one rep.

Jump Squat

Start by doing a regular squat and then jump up as explosively as you can when you rise up reaching for the ceiling. When you land, lower your body back into the squat position and continue. That's one rep.

Jump Lunge

Lunge forward with first leg. Land on heel then forefoot. Lower body by flexing knee and hip of front leg until knee of rear leg is almost in contact with floor then explode up by jumping into the same movement for the other leg. That's one rep.

Pull Ups

With palms facing away with a slightly wider than shoulder width grip, hang from an overhead bar and pull body up until chin elevates over the bar. Lower body until arms are fully extended. That's one rep.

Deadlift (Barbell & Dumbbell)

Squat down and grasp bar or dumbbells with shoulder width or slightly wider over hand or mixed grip. Lift bar or dumbbells by extending hips and knees to full extension. Pull shoulders back at top of lift. That's one rep.

Squats (Barbell & Dumbbell)

Bend knees forward while allowing hips to bend back behind, keeping back straight and knees pointed same direction as feet. Descend until knees are bent at 90 degrees. Extend knees and hips until legs are straight. Return to start position. That's one rep.

Step Ups (Barbell & Dumbbell)

Place foot of first leg on bench. Stand on bench by extending hip and knee of first leg and place foot of second leg on bench. Step down with second leg by flexing hip and knee of first leg. Return to original standing position by placing foot of first leg to floor. That's one rep.

Walking Lunges (Barbell & Dumbbell)

Lunge forward with first leg. Land on heel then forefoot. Lower body by flexing knee and hip of front leg until knee of rear leg is almost in contact with floor. Then step forward with other leg and repeat. That's one rep.

Wide Grip Lat Pull Downs

Sit down at machine. Grab overhead bar with wide grip. Sit with thighs under supports. Pull bar to upper chest. Return until arms and shoulders are fully extended.

Bench Press & Incline Bench Press(Barbell & Dumbbell)

Lie down on bench. Lower weight to mid-chest. Press weight upward until arms are extended. That's one rep.

For one arm incline bench press, elevate bench a few notches so the bench is inclined. Only hold weight in one of your arms. This will place more emphasis on your core stabilizers.

Bent Over Row (Barbell & Dumbbell)

Bend knees slightly and bend over with back almost parallel to the ground. Pull weight to upper waist. Return until arms are extended. That's one rep.

For the one arm dumbbell row, use the same form but just use weight in one arm.

Shoulder Press (Barbell & Dumbbell)

Press weight upward until arms are extended overhead. That's one rep.

Barbell Clean & Press

Grasp the bar with an overhand grip (both palms facing you) about shoulder width. Keeping your back straight and head facing forwards, deadlift the bar off the floor. Explosively drive the bar upwards through the hips and knees. As the bar reaches the thighs, simultaneously drop under the weight by bending at the knees. Reverse curl the bar up to rest on the shoulders by throwing your elbows underneath the bar and stand up straight. Then from the shoulders, push press the barbell up and over the head. Return the bar to the floor by performing the opposite set of movements. That's one rep.

Front Squat (Barbell & Dumbbell)

If using barbell, grasp barbell from rack with overhand open grip, slightly wider than shoulder width. Position barbell chest high with back arched. Place bar in front of shoulders with elbows placed forward as high as possible and finger under bar to each side With heels hip width or slightly wider, position feet outward at approximately 45°. Descend until knees and hips are fully bent or until thighs are parallel to floor. Knees travel outward in direction of toes. Extend knees and hips until legs are straight. Return to top position. That's one rep.

If using dumbbells, place dumbbells vertically and sit them on top of your shoulders. Follow same movement as described above.

Barbell Cleans

Stand over barbell with balls of feet positioned under bar pointing foward, hip width's apart or slightly wider. Squat down and grip bar with overhand grip slightly wider than shoulder width. Position shoulders over bar with back arched tightly. Arms are straight with elbows pointed along bar. Pull bar up off floor by extending hips and knees. As bar reaches knees vigorously raise shoulders while keeping barbell close to thighs. When barbell passes mid-thigh, allow it to contact thighs. Jump upward extending body. Shrug shoulders and pull barbell upward with arms allowing elbows to flex out to sides, keeping bar close to body. Aggressively pull body under bar, rotating elbows around bar. Catch bar on shoulders while moving into squat position. Hitting bottom of squat, stand up immediately. That's one rep.

Box Jumps

Stand in front of a stable box/bench or platform. Jump onto box and immediately back down to same position. That's one rep.

Dumbbell Bicep Curl To Overhead Shoulder Press

In one movement, curl dumbbell with palms facing away and then immediately rotate wrists and press weight overhead. That's one rep.

Underhand Chin Up

With palms facing towards the body with a shoulder width grip, hang from an overhead bar and pull body up until chin elevates over the bar. Lower body to until arms are fully extended. That's one rep.

One Arm Snatch

Pull dumbbell up off floor by extending hips and knees. As weight reaches knees back stays arched and maintains same angle to floor as in starting position. When weight passes knees vigorously raise shoulders while keeping bar as close to legs as possible. When weight passes upper thighs allow it to contact thighs. Jump upward extending body. Shrug shoulders and pull weight upward with arms. Aggressively pull body under dumbbell while moving into squat position. As soon as weight is caught with locked out arms in squat position, squat up into standing position with dumbbell overhead. That's one rep.

Barbell Hang Power Snatch

Start in the hang position with barbell in your hands, glutes pushed back, and ¼ bend at the waist. Snatch barbell up overhead by jumping upward extending body, shrug shoulders and pull barbell upward with arms allowing elbows to pull up to sides, keeping them over bar as long as possible. Aggressively pull body under bar. Catch bar at arm's length. That's one rep.

Barbell Push Press

Grasp barbell from rack with overhand grip, slightly wider than shoulder width. Position bar chest high with torso tight. Dip body by bending knees, hips and ankles slightly. Explosively drive upward with legs, driving barbell up off shoulders, vigorously extending arms overhead. Return to shoulders. That's one rep.

Dumbbell Reverse Lunge

Step back with one leg while bending supporting leg. Plant forefoot far back on floor. Lower body by flexing knee and hip of supporting leg until knee of rear leg is almost in contact with floor. Return to original standing position by extending hip and knee of forward supporting leg and return rear leg next to supporting leg. Repeat movement with opposite legs alternating between sides. That's one rep.

Dumbbell High Pull

Standing upright while gripping dumbbells with palms facing you, pull dumbbell up by jumping upward and flex elbows out to sides, pulling dumbbell up to neck height. Lower weight. That's one rep.

Dumbbell Arnold Press

Position two dumbbells in front of shoulders, palms facing body and elbows under wrists. Press dumbbells overhead and rotate wrists so palms face outward. Lower to front of shoulders in opposite pattern. That's one rep.

Barbell Upright Row

Grasp bar with shoulder width or slightly narrower overhand grip. Pull bar to neck with elbows leading. Allow wrists to flex as bar rises. Lower. That's one rep.

Barbell Power Clean & Jerk

Stand over barbell with balls of feet positioned under bar slightly wider apart than hip width. Squat down and grip bar with overhand grip slightly wider than shoulder width. Position shoulders over bar with back arched tightly. Arms are straight with elbows pointed along bar. Pull bar up off floor by extending hips and knees. As bar reaches knees vigorously raise shoulders while keeping barbell close to thighs. When barbell passes mid-thigh, allow it to contact thighs. Jump upward extending body. Shrug shoulders and pull barbell upward with arms allowing elbows to flex out to sides, keeping bar close to body. Aggressively pull body under bar, rotating elbows around bar. Catch bar on shoulders while moving into squat position. Hitting bottom of squat, stand up immediately. Inhale and position chest high with torso tight. Keeping pressure on heels, dip body by bending knees and ankles slightly. Explosively drive upward with legs, driving barbell up off shoulders. Drop body downward and split one foot forward and other backward as fast as possible while vigorously extending arms overhead. The split position places front shin vertical to floor with front foot flat on floor. The rear knee is slightly bent with rear foot positioned on toes. The bar should be positioned directly over ears at arms length with back straight. Push up with both legs. Position feet side by side by bringing front foot back part way and then rear foot forward. Lower barbell to shoulders. Then bend knees slightly and lower barbell to mid-thigh position.

For picture demonstrations with instructions of these exercises visit:

http://www.awakentheabswithin.com/awaken-the-abs-within-exercises/

Beginner Home Circuit Training For Fat Loss

Circuit training is great for fat loss because it keeps you constantly moving with minimal breaks. If you aren't a member of a gym or are just beginning at the gym, complete this workout program before moving on to the more advanced program to follow.

This program gives you a good aerobic workout by keeping your HR at an elevated state while also helping increase strength and muscle via the resistance-training portion. Rather than the traditional lift, rest, lift method. Circuit training is exercise #1 lift, exercise #2 lift, exercise #3 lift, etc. You only take minimal breaks by moving from one exercise to the next. It's intense and gets you fat loss results.

Since not everyone can afford to have a gym membership, I'm also including a fat loss circuit program that can be completed at home. If you don't have a pair of dumbbells, you can buy a cheap pair at Wal-Mart. If you don't want to buy them, use a bag of flour, a paint can, or some other household item as resistance.

Week 1-4 Fat Loss Home Workout Routine

This 4-week at home circuit program will rev up your metabolism, burn fat, and build lean muscle tissue.

Perform each exercise for 30 seconds. Complete as a circuit (finish one 30 second set and then move on to the next exercise). Do not rest between sets. Take a 1 minute break between each completed circuit. Complete 3 circuits. Perform this routine 3 days per week for 4 weeks.

Exercise	Circuit	Time	Reps	Weight
Jumping Jacks	1	30 sec		
	2	30 sec		
	3	30 sec		
High Knees	1	30 sec		
	2	30 sec		
	3	30 sec		
Dumbbell Squat and Press	1	30 sec		
	2	30 sec		
	3	30 sec		
Push Up	1	30 sec		
	2	30 sec		
	3	30 sec		
Lunges	1	30 sec/leg		
	2	30 sec/leg		
	3	30 sec/leg		
Chair Dip	1	30 sec		
	2	30 sec		

	3	30 sec		
Crunch	1	30 sec		
	2	30 sec		
	3	30 sec		

Week 5-8 Fat Loss Home Workout Routine

This intermediate 4-week routine will continue to blast that annoying fat and tone your entire body. You can do this workout in the comfort of your own home.

Perform each exercise for 45 seconds. Complete as a circuit (finish one 45 second set and then move on to the next exercise). Do not rest between sets. Take a 1 minute break between each completed circuit. Complete 3 circuits. Perform this routine 4 days per week for 4 weeks.

Exercise	Circuit	Time	Reps	Weight
High Knees	1	45 sec		
	2	45 sec		
	3	45 sec		
Mountain Climbers	1	45 sec		
	2	45 sec		
	3	45 sec		

Burpees	1	45 sec		
	2	45 sec		
	3	45 sec		
Dumbbell Squat and Press	1	45 sec		
	2	45 sec		
	3	45 sec		
Dumbbell Renegade Row	1	45 sec		
	2	45 sec		
	3	45 sec		
Lunges	1	45 sec/leg		
	2	45 sec/leg		
	3	45 sec/leg		
Kettlebell Swing	1	45 sec		
	2	45 sec		
	3	45 sec		
Plank	1	45 sec		
	2	45 sec		
	3	45 sec		

Side Plank	1	45 sec/side		
	2	45 sec/side		
	3	45 sec/side		

Week 9-12 Fat Loss Home Workout Routine

This more advanced 4-week routine will continue to torch the fat and tone your lean muscle tissue. More focus is placed on the core in this routine. You can do this workout in the comfort of your own home.

Perform each exercise for 60 seconds. Complete as a circuit (finish one 60 second set and then move on to the next exercise). Do not rest between sets. Take a 1 minute break between each completed circuit. Complete 3 circuits. Perform this routine 5 days per week for 4 weeks.

Exercise	Set	Time	Reps	Weight
Jump Rope	1	60 sec		
	2	60 sec		
	3	60 sec		
Mountain Climbers On Swiss Ball	1	60 sec		
	2	60 sec		
	3	60 sec		
Burpees	1	60 sec		

	2	60 sec		
	3	60 sec		
One Legged Dumbbell Squat	1	60 sec/leg		
	2	60 sec/leg		
	3	60 sec/leg		
Dumbbell Renegade Row + Side Plank	1	60 sec		
	2	60 sec		
	3	60 sec		
Lunges	1	60 sec/leg		
	2	60 sec/leg		
	3	60 sec/leg		
Kettlebell Swing	1	60 sec		
	2	60 sec		
	3	60 sec		
Lying Hip Raises	1	60 sec		
	2	60 sec		
	3	60 sec		
V-Ups	1	60 sec		

	2	60 sec		
	3	60 sec		

Week 13-15 Fat Loss Home Workout Routine

Exercise	Circuit	Reps	Weight	Rest
Burpees	1	12		25 sec
	2	12		25 sec
	3	12		25 sec
	4	12		25 sec
Inverted Row	1	12		25 sec
	2	12		25 sec
	3	12		25 sec
	4	12		25 sec
Ab Wheel	1	15		10 sec
	2	15		10 sec
	3	15		10 sec
	4	15		10 sec
Jump Squat	1	10		25 sec

	2	10		25 sec
	3	10		25 sec
	4	10		25 sec
Jump Lunges	1	10		25 sec
	2	10		25 sec
	3	10		25 sec
	4	10		25 sec
Pull Ups	1	10		10 sec
	2	10		10 sec
	3	10		10 sec
	4	10		10 sec

More Advanced Resistance Training Full Body Workout

The full body workout covered in this program has been strategically designed to create a metabolic response in the body that will increase your body's resting metabolic rate (RMR), burn more calories, and release more fat burning hormones and enzymes. The metabolic response of this program far exceeds workouts that strictly target 1-2 muscle groups per workout or just doing 100% cardio.

Studies show that your RMR can increase for 1-2 DAYS after large muscle group workouts. Compare this increase in RMR to a RMR increase of only 1-2 hours if you just followed a cardio only program. Don't get me wrong, cardio is important and will be a part of your program, but it won't be the biggest piece of the puzzle.

If you think the most effective exercises to awaken the abs within are crunches and sit ups, guess again. I can't say this enough, to find your abs; you need to burn off the belly fat. In order to burn the belly fat you need to perform exercises that burn the most calories. Ab specific exercises don't burn enough calories to really bring out your abs. There is no such thing as spot fat reduction. That's why you should be focusing your lifting program on compound multi-muscle exercises that burn the most calories when completing a rep and release the necessary fat burning hormones and enzymes. These compound exercises also use the abs to stabilize the body when performing the move.

I'm referring to the following compound/multi-joint exercises:

- Clean & Press
- Deadlifts
- Dips
- Lunges
- Presses
- Pull-Downs
- Pull-Ups/Chin-Ups
- Push-Ups
- Rows
- Snatches

- Squats
- Step-Ups
- Swings

What Is A Compound/Multi-Joint Exercise?

Most exercises can be classified as either a multi-joint or single joint exercise. The big difference is multi-joint exercises recruit more than one muscle at a time while single-joint exercises tend to isolate only one muscle for the majority of the lift (although most single-joint exercises do use other muscles, just to a much smaller degree). So by recruiting more muscles you tend to burn more calories and release more fat burning hormones.

For example, a leg extension on a leg extension machine locks in the leg thereby isolating one muscle group (quadriceps). This would be classified as a single-joint isolation exercise. Compare this move with a barbell squat. During a barbell squat, your body recruits many different muscle groups including the quadriceps, hamstrings, glutes, core, etc. Which one do you think uses more energy to complete a rep?

Multi-Joint Exercises vs. Single-Joint Exercise

There's no question that multi-joint exercises require a higher workload to complete than single-joint exercises. What do I mean by workload?

Work (W) = Force (F) * Distance (D)

Force = the amount of weight * # of reps * # of sets

Distance = the distance the weight is moved (in feet)

Lets apply the above formula to two different exercises so we can see which exercise has a higher workload to complete:

Leg Extension vs. Barbell Clean & Press

Work Load of Exercise #1:

Leg Extension (140 lbs x 12 reps x 3 sets)

Force = 140 x 12 x 3 = 5,040

Distance = 0.5 feet

Total Work Load Via Barbell Front Shoulder Raise= 5,040 * 0.5 = **2,520 lbs/foot**

Work Load of Exercise #2:

Barbell Clean & Press (135 lbs barbell x 12 reps x 3 sets)

Force = 135 x 12 x 3 = 4,860

Distance = 4 feet

Total Work Load Via Barbell Clean & Press = 4,860 * 4 = **19,440 lbs/foot**

As you can clearly see, selecting the right kind of multi-joint exercises is key.

Although you're lifting similar weight and completing the same amount of sets and reps, the Barbell Clean & Press takes over **7 times more work** to complete (in the same amount of time) than the Leg Extension.

To sum it up:

Higher workloads = More calorie burn + Better hormonal response + Greater metabolic response

Higher workloads are accomplished by focusing on multi-joint exercises that recruit numerous different muscles (thus allowing you to lift more weight) and require the weight to be moved in a longer range of motion (greater distance).

You will notice many of the exercises in the full body workout program are classified as higher workload exercises.

Free Weights vs. Machines?

Free weights (dumbbells/barbells/kettlebells, etc) are far more effective than machines. Machines lock in the movement/range of motion, thus taking away the need of your stabilizer muscles to perform the exercise correctly. Since the machine is locked in, it's essentially performing a good portion of the work for you. Don't believe me? Try completing a barbell squat in a locked in smith machine (a machine that locks in the bar so the weight can only move up and down) and then use the same weight (be careful) using a free weight barbell squat. Do you notice a difference in difficulty? What about overall muscle recruitment? I bet you struggled to lift the same weight and felt a greater overall muscle burn when you did the free weight barbell squat. This is because the movement is not controlled which causes your body to recruit all of it's stabilizer muscles on top of the major muscle groups to properly perform the movement.

However, I do believe machines are useful under the right circumstances. If you are new to lifting weights, and are not privy to the proper range of motion of certain exercises, I recommend you start with the machines. This is strictly for safety reasons. Once you get comfortable with the range of motion and the feeling in the muscle, move on to free weights. Machines can also be good to break out of plateaus if you've noticed your results have hit a wall.

Try to maintain an 80/20 breakdown of free weights-to-machines for best results.

Also note: I classify non-fixed cable machines to be free weights, as the range of motion is not fixed. These would include, lat pull down, row, and cable cross machines.

Full Body Multi-Joint Fat Burning Workout

If you're more experienced you can skip the beginner workout discussed earlier and go straight to the intermediate program. Be sure to stretch for 5-10 minutes after you complete the workouts.

Intermediate Program

Week 1-4 Workout Schedule

Day	Mon	Tues	Wed	Thurs	Fri	Sat	Sun
Week 1	A	HIIT	B	OFF	C	OFF	HIIT or Steady Pace
Week 2	A	HIIT	B	HIIT or Steady Pace	C	OFF	A
Week 3	HIIT	B	HIIT or Steady Pace	C	HIIT	A	OFF
Week 4	B	HIIT	C	HIIT or Steady Pace	A	OFF	B

Workout A

To be completed in a circuit. Complete A1, A2, A3, and A4 sequentially, resting for 30 seconds between exercises, then rest for 60 seconds after the circuit. Repeat 1 more time. Then complete circuit B the same way as indicated.

Complete 5-10 minute Warmup			
Exercise (Circuits)	**Circuits**	**Reps**	**Rest**
A1. Barbell Deadlifts	2	12	30 sec
A2. Barbell Squats	2	12	30 sec
A3. Dumbbell Step Ups	2	12/leg	30 sec
A4. Dumbbell Walking Lunges	2	12/leg	60 sec
Complete Circuit A Twice, Rest 90 seconds, Move on to Circuit B			
B1. Wide Grip Lat Pull Down	2	12	30 sec
B2. Barbell Bench Press	2	12	30 sec
B3. Barbell Bent Over Rows	2	12	30 sec
B4. Two-Arm Kettlebell or Dumbbell Swing	2	12	60 sec
Complete Circuit B Twice, Rest 90 seconds, Move on to 10-15 Minutes of Ab Training			

Workout B

Complete 5-10 minute Warmup			
Exercise (Circuits)	**Circuits**	**Reps**	**Rest**
A1. Dumbbell Squats	2	12	30 sec
A2. Dumbbell Deadlifts	2	12	30 sec
A3. Barbell Walking Lunges	2	12/leg	30 sec
A4. Barbell Step Ups	2	12/leg	60 sec
Complete Circuit A Twice, Rest 90 seconds, Move on to Circuit B			
B1. One Arm Dumbbell Row	2	12/arm	30 sec
B2. Dumbbell Bench Press	2	12	30 sec
B3. Seated Dumbbell Shoulder Press	2	12	30 sec
B4. One-Arm Kettlebell or Dumbbell Swing	2	12/arm	60 sec
Complete Circuit B Twice, Rest 90 seconds, Move on to 10-15 Minutes of Ab Training			

Workout C

Complete 5-10 minute Warmup			
Exercise (Circuits)	**Circuits**	**Reps**	**Rest**
A1. Barbell Walking Lunges	2	12/leg	30 sec
A2. Dumbbell Step Ups	2	12/leg	30 sec
A3. Dumbbell Squats	2	12	30 sec
A4. Barbell Deadlifts	2	12	60 sec
Complete Circuit A Twice, Rest 90 seconds, Move on to Circuit B			
B1. Barbell Bench Press	2	12	30 sec
B2. One-Arm Kettlebell or Dumbbell Swing	2	12/arm	30 sec
B3. Wide Grip Lat Pulldown	2	12	30 sec
B4. Seated Dumbbell Shoulder Press	2	12	60 sec
Complete Circuit B Twice, Rest 90 seconds, Move on to 10-15 Minutes of Ab Training			

Intermediate-Advanced Program

Week 5-8 Workout Schedule

Day	Mon	Tues	Wed	Thurs	Fri	Sat	Sun
Week 1	A	HIIT	B	OFF	C	OFF	HIIT or Steady Pace
Week 2	A	HIIT	B	HIIT or Steady Pace	C	OFF	A
Week 3	HIIT	B	HIIT or Steady Pace	C	HIIT	A	OFF
Week 4	B	HIIT	C	HIIT or Steady Pace	A	OFF	B

Workout A

To be completed in a circuit. Complete A1, A2, A3, and A4 sequentially, resting for 25 seconds between exercises, then rest for 50 seconds after the circuit. Repeat 2 more times. Then complete circuit B the same way as indicated.

Complete 5-10 minute Warmup			
Exercise (Circuits)	**Circuits**	**Reps**	**Rest**
A1. Barbell Clean & Press	3	6	25 sec
A2. Barbell Front Squat	3	12	25 sec
A3. Jump Squats	3	12	25 sec
A4. Jump Lunges	3	12	50 sec
Complete Circuit A Twice, Rest 90 seconds, Move on to Circuit B			
B1. Wide Grip Pull-ups (use assisted pullup machine if can't do more than 6)	3	Till failure	25 sec
B2. Barbell Bent Over Rows	3	12	25 sec
B3. Barbell Cleans	3	6	25 sec
B4. One-Arm Dynamic Kettlebell or Dumbbell Swing	3	12/arm	50 sec
Complete Circuit B Twice, Rest 90 sec, Move on to 10-15 min of Ab Training			

Workout B

Complete 5-10 minute Warmup			
Exercise (Circuits)	**Circuits**	**Reps**	**Rest**
A1. Barbell Front Squats	3	12	25 sec
A2. Barbell Clean & Press	3	6	25 sec
A3. Box Jumps	3	12	25 sec
A4. Jump Lunges	3	12/leg	50 sec
Complete Circuit A Twice, Rest 90 seconds, Move on to Circuit B			
B1. One Arm Dumbbell Row	3	12/arm	25 sec
B2. One Arm Incline Dumbbell Bench Press	3	12/arm	25 sec
B3. Dumbbell Bicep Curl To Overhead Shoulder Press	3	12/arm	25 sec
B4. One-Arm Dynmaic Kettlebell or Dumbbell Swing	3	12/arm	50 sec
Complete Circuit B Twice, Rest 90 seconds, Move on to 10-15 Minutes of Ab Training			

Workout C

Complete 5-10 minute Warmup			
Exercise (Circuits)	**Circuits**	**Reps**	**Rest**
A1. Barbell Walking Lunges	3	12/leg	25 sec
A2. Barbell Step Ups	3	12/leg	25 sec
A3. Dumbbell Squats & Press	3	12	25 sec
A4. Barbell Deadlifts	3	12	50 sec
Complete Circuit A Twice, Rest 90 seconds, Move on to Circuit B			
B1. Barbell Incline Bench Press	3	12	25 sec
B2. One-Arm Dynamic Kettlebell or Dumbbell Swing	3	12/arm	25 sec
B3. Underhand Chin Up (use assisted pullup machine if can't do more than 6)	3	Till Failure	25 sec
B4. One Arm Snatch	3	12/arm	50 sec
Complete Circuit B Twice, Rest 90 seconds, Move on to 10-15 Minutes of Ab Training			

Intermediate-Advanced Program

Week 9-12 Workout Schedule

Day	Mon	Tues	Wed	Thurs	Fri	Sat	Sun
Week 1	A	HIIT	B	OFF	C	OFF	HIIT or Steady Pace
Week 2	A	HIIT	B	HIIT or Steady Pace	C	OFF	A
Week 3	HIIT	B	HIIT or Steady Pace	C	HIIT	A	OFF
Week 4	B	HIIT	C	HIIT or Steady Pace	A	OFF	B

Complexes

These workouts consist of complexes. There are no breaks between exercises during a complex. You don't even get to drop the barbell or dumbbell between exercises. Therefore, select a weight for your most difficult exercise that you can lift for the prescribed rep count. You will use this weight for the entire complex as the weight won't leave your hands. If you aren't sweating after these workouts…you're not alive!

To be completed in a circuit. Complete A1, A2, A3, and A4 sequentially, no rest between exercises (keep weight in your hand). Rest for 120 seconds after the circuit. Repeat 3 more times. Then complete circuit B the same way as indicated.

Workout A - Complexes

Complete 5-10 minute Warmup			
Exercise (Complexes)	**Circuits**	**Reps**	**Rest**
A1. Barbell Hang Power Snatch	4	8	0 sec
A2. Barbell Push Press	4	8	0 sec
A3. Barbell Deadlift	4	8	0 sec
A4. Barbell Bent Over Row	4	8	120 sec
Complete Complex 4 Times, Rest 120 seconds, Move on to Complex B			
B1. Two Arm Dumbbell or Kettlebell Swing	4	10	0 sec
B2. Dumbbell Reverse Lunge	4	10/leg	0 sec
B3. Dumbbell Front Squat	4	10	0 sec
B4. Dumbbell Shoulder Press	4	10	120 sec
Complete Complex B 4 Twice, Rest 90 seconds, Move on to 10-15 Minutes of Ab Training			

Workout B - Complexes

Complete 5-10 minute Warmup			
Exercise (Complexes)	**Circuits**	**Reps**	**Rest**
A1. Dumbbell High Pull	4	10	0 sec
A2. Dumbbell Arnold Press	4	10	0 sec
A3. Dumbbell Bent Over Two Arm Row	4	10	0 sec
A4. Dumbbell Step Ups	4	10/leg	120 sec
Complete Complex 4 Times, Rest 120 seconds, Move on to Complex B			
B1. Barbell Squat	4	10	0 sec
B2. Barbell Deadlift	4	10/leg	0 sec
B3. Barbell Bent Over Row	4	10	0 sec
B4. Barbell Push Press	4	10	120 sec
Complete Complex B 4 Times, Rest 90 seconds, Move on to 10-15 Minutes of Ab Training			

Workout C - Complexes

Complete 5-10 minute Warmup			
Exercise (Complexes)	**Circuits**	**Reps**	**Rest**
A1. Barbell Upright Rows	4	8	0 sec
A2. Barbell Power Clean & Jerk	4	8	0 sec
A3. Barbell Deadlift	4	8	0 sec
A4. Barbell Jump Squats	4	8	120 sec
Complete Complex 4 Times, Rest 120 seconds, Move on to Complex B			
B1. Dumbbell Shoulder Press	4	10	0 sec
B2. Dumbbell Two Arm Bent Over Row	4	10	0 sec
B3. Dumbbell Front Squat	4	10	0 sec
B4. Dumbbell Jump Lunges	4	10/leg	120 sec
Complete Complex B 4 Twice, Rest 90 seconds, Move on to 10-15 Minutes of Ab Training			

There you have it. Including the initial 15-week beginner workouts, I've just provided you with 30 weeks of full body workouts. The 30 weeks are broken out into 4-week phases. This will ensure your body doesn't get used to any program, thus reducing the risk of plateauing.

Combine these workouts with a solid nutrition plan (as outlined earlier in this book) and you'll be well on your way to awakening the abs within. Oh yeah, what about your ab training? Keep reading.

Your Abdominals

When you ask most people what their vision of a healthy and fit body is, most reply "chiseled six pack abs" (males) or "a flat and tight stomach" (females). Every year fitness marketers thrive on this desire with the next big gadget that will develop your abs in the least amount of time. As you've learned throughout this program, awakening your abs is about lowering you body fat % to a low enough level to clearly see your abdominal muscles. You can follow this abdominal training program to the T but if you don't correct your diet first and employ all the strategies listed earlier, you will not get the results you're looking for. Once again, Abs are made in the kitchen, not in the gym. Your abs are strengthened and sculpted in the gym.

A Six Pack Is Great, But Can I Get An Eight-Pack?

This depends on your body type. If you have a long back and short legs you may be able to achieve an eight-pack look. However, if you have a short back and long legs you may only be able to achieve a six pack or four pack look. Don't look at this as being a bad thing. Remember, if you can get your body fat low enough to even see your abs, you're in the elite 3-4% class of the overall population. Don't get caught up in genetics.

The fat that accumulates below the bellybutton can create the most challenge. In men, this is simply because body fat tends to store itself more readily in the lower ab region (below the bellybutton) as opposed to the upper ab region closer to the sternum. This is because it's essentially the center of gravity. Getting rid of this last bit of belly fat is mainly about your diet. Follow the secrets in this book and you can torch this lower body fat and create the six pack look.

Abs Are A Unique Muscle

Unlike other muscles where they grow bigger when you work them out, the abs don't work that way. When you workout your abs, the goal is to make them flat, chiseled, and defined. Due to there proximity to the heart and lungs, abs are known as a rapidly re-oxidizing muscle group meaning you don't need long breaks to rest as they quickly get blood back to the muscle after you train them. So you only need a few seconds rest between sets before you attack them with intensity again.

I'm going to touch on this stuff in more detail, but my advice to get the most out of your ab workouts is to use as many different variables as you can. Change weights, reps, tempo, frequency, sets, volume, types of exercises, and angles you're hitting your abs.

Before we get into the ab exercises, it's important to understand the function of your abs to ensure you train safely and reduce the risk of any potential injury.

Functions Of The Abs

Rectus Abdominis (better known as the upper and lower abs) – This is the most prominent and noticeable area of the abs. It's the area that will give you the six pack effect. It runs vertically between your pubis and the ribs. The six pack effect is created by one vertical line down the middle and three horizontal lines across the rectus abdominis (called tendinous sheath). The rectus abdominis functions to help flex the spine when narrowing the space between the ribs and the pelvis. Therefore, to work the rectus abdominis, you need to narrow the angle between your ribs and pelvis by crunching the upper or lower body.

Obliques (External & Internal) – The obliques are located on each side of the rectus abdominis. The muscle fibers run vertically on a diagonal from the lower ribs to the pelvis. It forms the letter "V". Ever hear of the V-cut? The obliques function to help support and flexion of the spine, torso rotation, and stabilize the abdomen.

Transversus Abdominis – This is the deep layer of abdominal muscle. It wraps around the torso from the ribs to the pelvis, front to back. The muscle fibers run horizontally. This part of the abs helps with exhaling air from the lungs and can stabilize the spine. Great for maximizing core strength and giving you the look of having a smaller waist (you use your transversus abdominis when you suck in your stomach).

SIDE NOTE: Role of the Hip Flexors – Although not an official muscle of the abs, hip flexors do come into play a lot when exercising the abs. Certain 'ab exercises' can actually pull in more usage of the hips rather than the abs. In addition to sculpting your abs, for balance and safety, you should also focus on developing an overall strong core, including the hip flexors and lower back muscles.

Abdominal Training Program Framework

Abdominal Training Tips:

1. Strict/Proper Form

Proper form is key to safely recruit all the necessary muscle fibers to build strong and sculpted abs. This tip is often overlooked in the gym. To properly develop your abs, you should be maintaining proper posterior pelvic tilt. I know…woah, what does that mean? Well look at it this way, when you're lying on the floor to do a crunch or hanging to do a leg/knee raise, is your back arched or rounded? Take note next time. If your back is arched, your pelvis has an anterior pelvic tilt (the opposite form you should be using). Remove the arch out of your back and rotate your pelvis to the floor. This creates a proper posterior pelvic tilt which is optimal to work your abs. By properly rounding your back, you place more emphasis on the abs and less emphasis on the hip flexors. When I first started working out, I always did hanging leg raises the wrong way. I always felt my hip flexors working more than my abs. The position of my pelvic region was the problem. And another thing, don't forget to curl your pelvis towards your upper body or vice versa! You'll notice this will make the exercise more difficult but you'll be placing much more stress on the abs.

2. Focus – The Mind Muscle Connection

Always, always, always focus on feeling the abdominals being worked. This tip is actually true for any type of resistance training. If you don't feel the muscle (abs) being worked, you potentially aren't placing the stress on the right muscle and could be creating an environment for injury. Always ensure the contraction is being felt in the area you are training. In this case, we're focusing on the abs.

3. Breathing – The Importance of Exhaling During Contraction

Every time you are contracting the muscle you should be pulling your belly button in toward your spine and exhale all the air out of your system. I'm not just talking about a quick breathe out. I want you breathing out as much carbon dioxide as possible. This will place maximum contraction on your abdominal region. Ever notice when you have a cold and can't control your coughing your abs actually hurt. This is because you're contracting your abs every time you cough. Lets try this quick exercise. Take off your shirt and stand in front of a mirror (preferably in private). Now open your mouth and breath out as much air as possible. Notice how you have to contract your abs to do this? You should be doing this every single rep when you are training your abs. Always flex!

4. Abdominal Symmetry – Hit All Parts of the Abdominals (including lower back)

To really develop the kind of six pack magazine cover look, you need to work all areas of the abdominals including the lower back. The lower back will also be worked via the full body exercises. Other areas of the abs include:

Rectus Abdominis (you may think you can isolate the 'upper' or 'lower' abs but you're really activating the entire region when you crunch the lower or upper body. However, it is very beneficial to work your abs in various directions and angles.)

Transverse Abdominus

Internal & External Obliques

The training workouts in this program will train all areas of the abs to give you the symmetrical six pack ab look.

Also be sure to complete the most difficult exercises first when you have the most energy.

5. Controlled Tempo - Quality vs. Quantity

It's more about feeling the abs contracting and tightening rather than using momentum and speed to get you through more reps. Allow your abs to do the work in a slow and controlled manner. Take momentum out of the equation. Every quality rep counts. The others are just a waste and can cause injury. Quality will bring the definition. Also ensure you're not pulling your head forward/or pulling your chin to your chest when doing crunches. I always recommend just placing your fingers on your ears. This will reduce the risk of pulling your head/neck out of alignment and creating injury.

6. Adding Resistance or Other Variables

Once you can complete the set amount of reps for the abs exercise in perfect form and tempo, add resistance in the form of a dumbbell, barbell plate, or resistance bands. Adding resistance can increase the cuts, definition, and separation in your abs. Or you can add other variables into the exercise such as balance and other core conditioning elements. For example, do a plank with one foot off the ground or with your forearms resting on a bosu or stability ball. Or you could hold the position for a longer period of time. Do the plank for 65 seconds rather than 60 seconds. Essentially always be changing the variables of your program, such as different weights, reps, tempo, frequency, sets, volume, types of exercises, and angles you're hitting the abs.

7. Don't Get Comfortable – Always Be Challenging Yourself

Don't become complacent and just complete the same routine in the same order, with the same resistance, etc. Your abdominals are like any other muscle. They will adapt and stop responding. This will quickly put the breaks on any progress. All training must be progressive. Change the order of the exercises, the resistance, the number of sets/reps, rest periods, tempo, and different angles.

8. Train Your Abs With a New Program For 10-15 Minutes After Most Workouts

Get into the habit of training your abs for 10-15 minutes after most workouts. If you run out of time or you are too tired to really train your abs hard, do the 10-15 minutes before your workout.

If you find you can keep training your abs, even after 15 straight minutes, you're probably not training them hard enough. As mentioned earlier, control every rep, contract your abs, and slow the tempo. After 10-15 straight minutes of this, you shouldn't be able to do anymore direct training. If you have a choice, do the ab routine after your full body workout since the abs stabilize the body. Therefore, if you really give your abs a solid workout before your full body program, your squats, deadlifts, etc. may suffer since your core is pre-exhausted. And remember to keep changing your routine.

Don't get stuck in a rut of doing the same exercises in the same way every time. Your body will adapt. Keep changing it up and keep the body guessing.

I directly train my abs 5-6 times per week but you can get away with 2-3 times.

9. Train With Intensity – Circuits or Supersets

Don't just end your workout day with a few lazy abs exercises. Train your abs with the same intensity as training your chest or legs. Also train your abs in circuits or supersets. Unlike other muscles that require a few minutes to recover between sets, your abs can quickly recover. Therefore you can increase the intensity by incorporating circuits and supersets into your abs training. This simply means you'll complete one set of a given abs exercise and then move into another abs exercise immediately without any rest. This is all laid out in the program. Feel the burn!

10. Hit Your Abs From All Angles

Variety is essential to abs training. For example, add decline leg raises to your routine rather than just doing flat bench leg raises. Also change the angle of the decline so you abs don't adapt. Always keep your abs guessing and wondering what's coming next.

Try completing the harder exercises earlier in your ab routine. These usually include any form of leg or lower body lifts.

11. Train Smart

Incorporate these training tips every time you attack your abs. There are multiple abs programs based on your current conditioning. If you're unsure of where you fit, start with the beginner program and work your way up. If you abs are not strong enough and you move into the intermediate or advanced program too quickly YOU WILL HURT YOURSELF. Always train smart by training safe. Six pack abs is a marathon, not a sprint.

My Two Favorite Ab Routines

I always change up my ab routine but here are my two all-time favorite ab circuits that I complete after my morning cardio or if I don't do cardio that day, after my workout. I always perform my ab routines with no breaks and in circuit format. This program usually takes me 10-15 minutes to complete.

My Favorite Sculpting & Defining Ab Routine 3 circuits (No Break)	
Exercise	**Rep Range**
A1. Hanging Leg Raise	15-20
A2. High Cable Rope Kneeling Crunch	20-30
A3. Decline Hip Raise	15-20
A4. Double Crunch	20-30
A5. High Cable Single Arm Kneeling Cable Crunch	20/arm
A6. V-Twist	20/side

My Favorite Strength & Conditioning Core Routine 3 Circuits (No Break)	
Exercise	Rep Range
A1. Hand Walk-Outs or Ab Roller	10-12
A2. Bosu and Medicine Ball Stability Plank	20-30
A3. Side Plank Drop Bend	12-15/side
A4. Side Plank Rotation Reach Through	12-15/side
A5. Inward Pike	10-12
A6. Back Extensions	12-15

Top 30 Abdominal Exercises

In addition to my favorite ab circuits mentioned above, here are the top 30 Abdominal Exercises to awaken the abs within broken out by section of abs – not order of effectiveness. For picture demonstrations with instructions visit:

http://www.awakentheabswithin.com/awaken-the-abs-within-exercises/

The level indicated in the brackets designates the degree of difficulty. Therefore you do not need to stick exclusively to the exact sample programs given. Just choose at least one exercise under each section that fits a level that you are currently at. Complete that exercise in the rep/duration as indicated in the sample program. Once you can comfortably complete the routine in level 1, you can move on to level 2, etc.

Strengthening Exercises:

Ab Wheel and/or Hand Walk Outs (Level 2-10)

Ab Wheel: Begin by kneeling on the floor, and hold both sides of the wheel. Roll the wheel forward, and lower your body as far as you can without arching your back. Then, use you abs to pull yourself back to the starting position. That's one rep.

Hand Walk Outs: Bend over at waist so your feet and hands are on the ground. Walk your hands out until your body is almost straight, then walk them back in. Keep the core engaged and contracted at all times. That's one rep.

Bosu and Medicine Ball Stability Plank and/or Swiss Ball Plank (Level 3-10)

Bosu and Medicine Ball Stability Plank: Bosu ball should be flat side towards the ground. Assume the plank position with forearms on bosu ball and feet on medicine ball. Keep core tight and hold for desired time.

Swiss Ball Plank: Assume the plank position with forearms on a swiss ball. Keep core tight and hold for desired time.

Renegade Dumbbell Row (Level 2-10)

Start in a push up position, gripping a pair of dumbbells. Pull one dumbbell up to your arm pit. Then repeat with the other arm. That's one rep.

Vacuums (Level 1-10)

Simply suck in your stomach and hold.

Oblique Exercises:

Alternating Elbow-To-Opposite-Knee Crunch (Level 1-10)

Lay on back with knees up. Crunch up and touch elbow to opposite knee. Repeat on other side. That's one rep.

Bicycle (Level 2-10)

Lay on back with legs straight. Crunch up, bring one elbow across the body while simultaneously bringing opposite knee towards elbow. Repeat other side. The leg portion mimics peddling a bike. That's one rep.

Breakdancer (Level 2-10)

Start in pushup position and quickly rotate core by bringing one leg to opposite side of body and then repeat the other side. Keep core tight throughout movement. That's one rep.

High Cable Single Arm Rope Elbow-To-Opposite Knee Crunch (Level 1-10)

Attach a rope attachment to a high cable pulley machine. Kneel on both knees while holding onto the rope attachment with one arm. Keeping your core tight, contract abs and curl pelvis to crunch toward the opposite knee. Repeat other side. That's one rep.

Seated Bar Twists (Level 1-10)

Sit on a bench with a light weighted bar on your shoulders similar to when you squat a barbell. Slowly twist torso to one side, pause, then twist back to center, pause, then twist to other side. That's one rep.

Side Plank (Level 2-10)

Lie on your side on a mat. Place forearm on mat under shoulder perpendicular to body. Place upper leg directly on top of lower leg and straighten knees and hips. Raise body upward by straightening waist so body is ridged. Hold. Repeat with opposite side.

Side Plank Drop Bend (Level 2-10)

Assume the side plank position then drop hips to the ground then bring back to the starting position. That's one rep. Complete reps and repeat other side.

Side Plank Reach-Through (Level 2-10)

Assume the side plank position then with your top arm extended over your body reach under your body, touch the ground behind you, and then return to starting position. That's one rep. Complete reps and repeat other side.

Swiss Ball Medicine Ball Or Cable Chop (Level 2-10)

While sitting on a swiss ball hold a medicine ball in both hands. Reach up and to one side of your body and then chop down to the opposite side. Similar movement to chopping a tree with an axe. That's one rep. Complete reps and repeat other side. You can also complete exercise by using a low cable pulley attachment.

Swiss Ball Side Twists (Level 3-10)

Lay on your side on top of swiss ball. With your feet in scissor position and against the wall bend at the waist down then simultaneously bend up and twist at the waist. That's one rep. Complete reps and repeat other side.

V-Twist (Level 2-10)

Sit on the ground with knees slightly bent. I find the obliques are activated more when the heels of my feet remain on the ground. With two hands, grasp a dumbbell/plate/medicine ball on both ends, rotate and touch down on one side of your body. Repeat on other side. That's one rep.

Rectus Abdominis:

Decline Hip Raise and/or Lying Hip Raise (Level 1-10)

Decline Hip Raise: Using a decline bench, grab the handles overhead and raise legs to a 90 degree angle (this is starting position). Perform a crunch by raising your legs towards your shoulders, thus closing the angle between your waist and shoulders. Lower legs back to 90 degrees. That's one rep.

Lying Hip Raise: While lying flat on the floor (hands can be under your glutes) raise legs up so there is a 90 degree angle formed at the hips (this is starting position). Thrust hips up in the air with legs reducing the angle between hips and shoulders. That's one rep.

Double Crunch and/or Weighted Crunch (Level 1-10)

Double Crunch: While lying on your back, place your heels on top of a bench. This is starting position. Perform a crunch while simultaneously curling your pelvis. Thus creating a double crunch. That's one rep.

Weighted Crunch: While lying on the floor holding a plate over your chest, perform a standard crunch. That's one rep.

Hanging Knee Raises (Level 3-10)

Hang from a pull up bar, place your elbows in straps, or use a roman chair machine. The key to this exercise is not to use momentum and ensure you round your back (don't arch it). The whole movement requires you to curl your pelvis. Don't just raise knees up and down (this is working the hip flexors more than the abs). Curl the pelvis with a rounded back when you raise your knees. Return knees to original position. That's one rep.

Hanging Leg Raises (Level 4-10)

Hang from a pull up bar, place your elbows in straps, or use a roman chair machine. The key to this exercise is not to use momentum and ensure you round your back (don't arch it). The whole movement requires you to curl your pelvis. Don't just raise legs up and down (this is working the hip flexors more than the abs). Curl the pelvis with a rounded back when you raise your slightly bent legs. Return legs to original position. That's one rep.

Half Burpee (Level 1-10)

Begin in a squat position with hands on the floor in front of you. Kick your feet back to a pushup position. Immediately return your feet to the squat position. That's one rep.

High Cable Rope Crunch (standing and kneeling) (Level 1-10)

Attached a rope attachment to a high cable pulley machine. Kneel on both knees while holding onto the rope attachment. Keeping your core tight, contract abs and curl pelvis to crunch toward the ground. That's one rep.

Inward Pike (Level 4-10)

Using a tricep dip bar, hold your body up with straight arms. This is the starting position. Now bring your hips up and in to form a pike. Lower your hips to starting position. That's one rep.

Mountain Climbers (Level 1-10)

Place hands on floor, slightly wider than shoulder width. While holding upper body in place, alternate leg positions by pushing hips up while immediately extending forward leg back and pulling rear leg forward under body, landing on both forefeet simultaneously. Once you bring in both knees, that's one rep.

Overhead Weighted Swiss Ball Crunch (Level 2-10)

With your lower back on a swiss ball, hold a plate over your chest. Perform a standard crunch. That's one rep.

Reverse Crunch (Level 1-10)

Lie on your back and bend your knees with your feet on the floor. Keeping your knees bent, raise your legs and curl your pelvis. Lower back to the floor. That's one rep.

Swiss Ball Knee Tuck Ins (Level 2-10)

Get in a push up position except put your feet on a swiss ball. Keeping your core tight, pull in your knees and then extend back out to the starting position. That's one rep.

V-Ups (Level 2-10)

Lay down on floor with hands overhead. Simultaneously raise straight legs and torso. Reach toward raised feet. Return to starting position. That's one rep.

Lower Back

Back Extension (Level 1-10)

Lay flat on the floor on your stomach. Extend your arms over your head like superman. In one motion lift your arms and legs up, pause, and lower. That's one rep.

Bird Dog (Level 2-10)

Get on your hands and knees (hands directly below your shoulders, knees directly below your hips). Slowly lift up your right leg backwards, and your left arm forwards (so they are parallel to the floor). Hold for 5 seconds and relax. Repeat with the opposite arm and leg. That's one rep.

Swiss Ball Reverse Hip Raise (Level 2-10)

Get in push up position but with your mid-section on top of a swiss ball. Your legs should be straight to start. Simply elevate legs until your body is straight. Lower legs. That's one rep.

What About Weighted Side Bends?

If you're looking for a bigger and blockier waist, do weighted side bends. If you're anything like me, you want the opposite look. You want a nice v-taper look of a smaller/tighter waist or the cobra look of a wide thick back and shoulders and a narrow tight waist.

When you do weighted side bends, you're building up the thickness of the muscle around the waist.

So if you want a tighter and smaller waist, leave out the side bends (with the exception of the swiss ball side twist which does not use weight and it's more of a rotation than a side bend).

Ab Exercise Program Samples

Here are a few ab exercise program samples. The higher the level, the higher the reps, sets, and more advanced exercises are chosen. You can choose any ab exercises you like.

Once you can complete the level with relative ease, you can proceed to the next level.

Level 1 Abs Program

1 circuit (No breaks)

Exercise	Rep Range
A1. Lying Hip Raises	10
A2. Double Crunch	15
A3. Alternating Elbow-To-Knee Crunch	10/side
A4. Plank on Floor	30 seconds
A5. Half Burpee	20

Level 2 Abs Program

1 circuit (No breaks)

Exercise	Rep Range
A1. Lying Hip Raises	15
A2. High Cable Rope Crunch (kneeling)	15
A3. Bicycle	15/side
A4. Mountain Climbers	40 (20/leg)
A5. Side Plank	45 sec

Level 3 Abs Program	
2 circuits (No breaks)	
Exercise	**Rep Range**
A1. Lying Hip Raises	15
A2. Weighted Crunch	15
A3. Bicycle	20/side
A4. Hand Walkouts	10
A5. Side Plank Drop Bends	12/side

Level 4 Abs Program	
2 circuits (No breaks)	
Exercise	**Rep Range**
A1. Hanging Knee Raises	15
A2. Renegade Dumbbell Row	6/side
A3. High Cable Single Arm Rope Elbow-To-Opposite Knee Crunch	15/side
A4. Ab Wheel	12
A5. Back Extensions	15

Level 5 Abs Program

2 circuits (No breaks)

Exercise	Rep Range
A1. Hanging Knee Raises	20
A2. Double Crunch	20
A3. Bicycle	20/side
A4. Swiss Ball Plank	45 sec
A5. Side Plank Reach-Through	12/side

Level 6 Abs Program

2 circuits (No breaks)

Exercise	Rep Range
A1. Hanging Leg Raises	12
A2. Decline Hip Raises	10
A3. Bicycle	20/side
A4. Breakdancer	15/side
A5. Bird Dog	12/side

Level 7 Abs Program	
2 circuits (No breaks)	
Exercise	**Rep Range**
A1. Hanging Leg Raises	15
A2. Reverse Crunch	20
A3. V-Ups	15
A4. Overhead Weighted Swiss Ball Crunch	15
A5. Seated Bar Twists	30

Level 8 Abs Program	
3 circuits (No breaks)	
Exercise	**Rep Range**
A1. Hanging Leg Raises	15
A2. Swiss Ball Knee Tuck Ins	15
A3. Bicycle	20/side
A4. Swiss Ball Cable Chop	20/side
A5. Swiss Ball Side Twists	12/side

Level 9 Abs Program	
3 circuits (No breaks)	
Exercise	**Rep Range**
A1. Hanging Leg Raises	20
A2. Hanging Knee Raises	25
A3. Bicycle	30/side
A4. Swiss Ball Side Twists	20/side
A5. Bosu and Medicine Ball Stability Ball Plank	60 sec

Level 10 Abs Program	
2 circuits (No breaks)	
Exercise	**Rep Range**
A1. Hanging Leg Raises	30
A2. Hanging Knee Raises	40
A3. High Cable Rope Crunch (Kneeling)	40
A4. Inward Pike	50
A5. V-Ups	40

Exercise Program Reminders

- A properly designed fat loss exercise program is comprised of a warm up, resistance training program, abdominal routine, and cardio program. The most important portion of this exercise program is the resistance-training portion.

- Try to focus the majority of your cardio program on HIIT routines. Complement this with steady state cardio to keep your program fresh.

- Focus on completing multi-joint compound exercises that move greater distances rather than single-joint exercises. The majority of your exercises should be higher workload exercises.

- Focus on using free weights more than machines (80-20 ratio)

- There is no such thing as spot reduction. You will burn off the most fat and calories during your full body lifting programs. The direct abdominal training is specifically intended to strengthen and sculpt your abs (not burn fat).

- Keep your workouts between 45-75 minutes.

- Lift weights 3-4 times per week (every other day) and cardio 2-3 times per week (can be during off lifting days). Take 1-2 days completely off from the gym.

- Try to train abs for 10-15 minutes after every workout.

- Train abs in a circuit format with no breaks. Keep it intense.

CONCLUSION

Thank you for reading Awaken The Abs Within. You are now equipped with all the information you need to transform your body. Keep this book close by. There is a lot of information contained in these pages. You may need to read it more than once to really absorb all the information.

Now…the next step is up to you.

You can have the best nutrition plan or exercise plan to lose belly fat and get a sexy tight stomach, but if you don't implement it and take it serious, it won't do you any good. Make the decision to change. Set short/long-term measurable and realistic goals to keep you accountable. A safe goal is to lose 1-2 pounds of fat every week. Implement this plan to get you to where you want to go. Stop talking about it and start taking action. Procrastination is the enemy. Don't put it off for another day.

Oh, and before you go…

Be sure to take a picture before you begin the program. You may not feel like it at the time, but I promise you, once you transform your body, you will want proof to show people how you looked before. I'm sure people won't believe your transformation without this picture.

I'd really appreciate it if you would e-mail me your testimonials and progress pictures. I love hearing about your success stories!

E-mail me at: brad@bradgouthrofitness.com

Welcome to the Elite 3-4% Abs Club. See you at the beach!

GET YOUR FREE BONUSES NOW!

Get more **FREE BONUSES** such as:

"9 Steps to: Healthy Eating" &

"5 Abdominal Fat Burning Foods"

by visiting: **http://www.awakentheabswithin.com/free-stuff/**

ABOUT

THE AUTHOR

• Owner of Brad Gouthro Fitness, a fitness, nutrition, and wellness publishing company specializing in helping people lose belly fat, build six pack abs, and living life to their greatest potential.

• Certified Personal Training Specialist (PTS) specializing in full body transformations, losing belly fat, getting six pack abs, and functional strength.

• Certified Nutrition & Wellness Specialist (NWS)

• Named finalist for Favorite Personal Trainer as voted by clients.

• Featured Cover Model of the "Lean Hybrid Muscle" fitness system program created by fitness gurus Elliot Hulse & Mike Westerdal.

Who am I and why am I the right person to write this book?

It's simple. As a certified personal trainer and nutrition and wellness specialist, I've been blessed with an uncontrollable passion for fitness, nutrition, and awakening the six pack abs within. It's in my DNA. Unfortunately the same passionate DNA didn't give me the golden ticket of also having a chiseled set of six pack abs.

My Journey

My journey began as a skinny kid who was very active in competitive sports. Even though I was a decent athlete (I still think I could be Peyton Manning's star Wide Receiver), I was always self-conscience of my ectomorph frame and pudgy stomach. Although it didn't look like it (maybe it was because I wore baggy clothes), I had a belly. Fortunately for me, I've always been high on self-improvement and enjoy the challenge of overcoming my weaknesses. This meant taking my Urkel-esque/fat belly frame and turning it into a strength. My initial attempts at working out produced very little results. It wasn't because I wasn't working hard. It was because I was very ignorant to the usage of proper training and diet methods to properly lose belly fat and build six pack abs. I quickly learned that transforming my body and awakening the abs within must be seen as a disciplined and structured marathon rather than a quick and unstructured sprint.

My Body Transformation

My body transformation began taking place after I hit a wall. I became so frustrated with my lack of physical progress that I had to take a step back and seek proper guidance. I consumed myself with everything related to fitness and nutrition (I still do today). Having an addictive personality, I researched everything I could about the in's and out's of building lean mass, losing belly fat, and sculpting six pack abs. After reading the right books and following the success stories of athletes that overcame the same challenges that I faced, I started implementing these best practices into my daily routines.

What Was The Result?

My close friends still make fun of my body today BUT it's because they can't believe the results of my body transformation. It's quite a different feeling being "chirped" by your buddies because YOU HAVE sculpted six pack abs, a v-shaped back, and chiseled arms.

So why should you follow my journey? I've been there, I've tried that. I've worked my butt off for very little results. It wasn't until I started implementing a structured fitness and, more importantly, solid nutrition plan into my lifestyle that I started to see my six pack abs. I understand what you're going through. That's why I know you'll appreciate the insights and best practices that I have to share. You only have one body. So treat it like your temple.

www.ingramcontent.com/pod-product-compliance
Lightning Source LLC
Chambersburg PA
CBHW060252290526
45789CB00001B/303